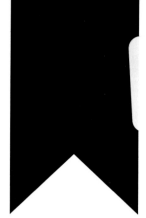

INTRODUCTION

to

CLINICAL RESEARCH

(For Medical Students, Residents, and Fellows)

Edited by

Tetyana L. Vasylyeva MD, PhD, DSc

Introduction to Clinical Research
First Aid for Sub-Specialty Boards and
Start-Up Research

Tetyana L. Vasylyeva MD, PhD, DSc

Hale Publishing, L.P.

1712 N. Forest St.

Amarillo, TX 79106-7017

806-376-9900

800-378-1317

www.iBreastfeeding.com

Library of Congress Control Number: 2011941953

ISBN-13: 978-0-9833075-9-4

Printing and Binding: Corley Printing Company, LLC

Table of Contents

Introduction and Overview 5

How to Address a Research Question 9

Matt Jeremiah T. Chua, MD

Christopher Giuliano, PharmD

Pradeep K. Selvaraj, MD, PhD

Clinical Study Designs Overview 19

Tetyana L. Vasylyeva, MD, PhD, DSc

The Institutional Review Board (IRB) and Health Insurance
Portability and Accountability Act (HIPAA) Regulations 37

Brian C. Weis, MD, PhD

Informed Consent to Participate in Research 49

Kathy Thomas, RN, CIP

Clinical Trials: Design and Monitoring 63

Craig Tipton, BBA

Majid Moridani, PharmD, PhD, DABCC, FACB

Clinical Research and Ethics.. 85

Osvaldo Regueria, MD

Walter Bridges, MD

Mubariz Naqvi, MD

A Basic Protocol 99

James K. Luce, MD

Candace A. Myers, PhD

Data Collection.. 105

Paul Tullar, MD

Robert P. Kauffman, MD

Introductory Statistics for Clinicians 109

Majid Moridani, PharmD, PhD, DABCC, FACB

Rajiv Balyan, DVM, MSc

Data Fraud and Authorship.. 141

Vinod K. Sethi, MD

Advice on Writing a Research Grant................................... 151

Candace A. Myers, PhD

The NIH Scientific Review and Ten Commandments for Grant
Success 163

Golder N. Wilson, MD, PhD

Industry and Philanthropy 177

Michael E. Okogbo, MD, MBA

Scientific Presentations.. 185

E.F. Luckstead, MD

Roger D. Smalligan, MD, MPH

Writing for Scientific Publication 195

Candace A. Myers, PhD

How to Survive and Thrive in the Peer Review Process.............. 205

Kathleen Kendall-Tackett, PhD, IBCLC, FAPA

References 217

Index... 227

Editor Bio 231

List of Contributors

Balyan, Rajiv, DVM, MSc
Doctoral student
Pharmaceutical Sciences
School of Pharmacy
Texas Tech University Health Sciences Center

Bridges, Walter, MD
Associate Professor
Department of Pediatrics
Texas Tech University Health Sciences Center

Chua, Matt Jeremiah T., MD
Assistant Professor
Department of Internal Medicine
Texas Tech University Health Sciences Center

Giuliano, Christopher, PharmD
Assistant Clinical Professor
Wayne State University
Eugene Applebaum College of Pharmacy and
Health Sciences
Clinical Specialist Internal Medicine
St. John Health System

Kauffman, Robert P., MD
Professor
Regional Chair (Amarillo, TX)
Department of Obstetrics and Gynecology
Texas Tech University Health Sciences Center

Kendall-Tackett, Kathleen, PhD, IBCLC, FAPA
Clinical Associate Professor
Department of Pediatrics
Texas Tech University Health Sciences Center

Luce, James K., MD
Retired Medical Director
Don and Sybil Harrington Cancer Center

Luckstead, E.F., MD
Professor
Department of Pediatrics
Texas Tech University Health Sciences Center

Moridani, Majid, PharmD, PhD, DABCC, FACB
Associate Professor
Department of Medicine
National Jewish Health
Denver, Colorado

Myers, Candace A., PhD
Assistant Professor
Clinical Research Unit
Texas Tech University Health Sciences Center

Naqvi, Mubariz, MD
Professor
Department of Pediatrics
Texas Tech University Health Sciences Center

Okogbo, Michael, MD, MBA
Associate Professor
Scott & White/Texas A&M College of Medicine,
Temple, TX
Former:
Department of Pediatrics
Texas Tech University Health Sciences Center

Regueria, Osvaldo, MD
Associate Professor
Department of Pediatrics
Texas Tech University Health Sciences Center

Selvaraj, Pradeep K., MD, PhD
Chief Resident
Department of Internal Medicine
Texas Tech University Health Sciences Center

Sethi, Vinod K., MD
Associate Professor
Department of Pediatrics
Texas Tech University Health Sciences Center

Smalligan, Roger D., MD, MPH
Associate Professor
Regional Chair (Amarillo)
Department of Internal Medicine
Texas Tech University Health Sciences Center

Thomas, Kathy, RN, CIP
Director
Texas Tech University Health Sciences Center
Amarillo IRB
Texas Tech University Health Sciences Center

Tipton, Craig, BBA
Department of Pharmaceutical Sciences
School of Pharmacy
Texas Tech University Health Sciences Center

Tullar, Paul E., MD, FACOG
Assistant Professor
Department of Obstetrics and Gynecology
Texas Tech University Health Sciences Center

Vasylyeva, Tetyana L., MD, PhD, DSc
Professor
Department of Pediatrics
Texas Tech University Health Sciences Center

Weiss, Brian C., MD, PhD
Associate Professor
Department of Internal Medicine
Texas Tech University Health Sciences Center

Wilson, Golder N., MD, PhD
Professor of Pediatrics
Professor of Obstetrics & Gynecology
Texas Tech University Health Sciences Center
KinderGenome Pediatric Genetics, Dallas

Introduction and Overview

*"If we knew what we were doing,
it wouldn't be called research, would it?"*
Albert Einstein

Dear Reader:

If you are reading this book, it means that you have a curious mind and want to advance medical science in its mission to protect the healthy and cure the sick. Our goal is to help you get started.

Medicine has always been evolving. Tremendous progress was made in the last few decades. We now know much more about genes and epigenetics, therapeutic cancer interventions, and cardiovascular disease prevention. We are able to take care of very low birth weight babies and challenge the slow destruction caused by diabetes. Unfortunately, there is still much we do not know, and there are many patients who live with the hope of a future cure. You are their hope.

Medical science can be divided into "bench research" or basic science, "translational research" or research that brings basic science to the clinic, and "clinical research," which directly involves human subjects. This book focuses on clinical research only.

Before you can implement your new clinical ideas in humans, you need to learn the history of the process and understand the rules and regulations that protect human subjects. Let us guide you over some of the hurdles on this challenging, but rewarding road.

The objective of this book is to provide healthcare trainees and professionals with practical, comprehensive, and contemporary approaches to clinical research. The book will be useful for anyone wishing to better understand modern research-based literature and for those who are planning to conduct their own research. We will focus each chapter on a key clinical research topic. We will discuss study designs, study monitoring, and which design fits certain research questions. Chapters will describe rules and regulations, which must be followed when conducting clinical research, including discussions of the Institutional Review Board, informed consent, and Health Insurance Portability and Accountability Act (HIPAA). The reader will be introduced to clinical trials and research ethics, data management, and the basic tools used in biostatistics. Individual chapters will discuss data fraud and authorship concerns. Readers will learn grant writing tips and how to find funding from the National Institutes of Health (NIH), industry, and private foundations. The final chapters will be dedicated to scientific presentations, research article writing skills, and how to manage the peer-review process.

We hope the book will provide paradigms for conducting state-of-the-art clinical research and open the horizons for future advances in medicine.

The inspiration for the book came from our students, residents, and young colleagues, who are very enthusiastic in pursuing research and moving the boundaries of medical knowledge forward. This book would never have been written without the strong support of Texas Tech University Health Sciences Center and the Clinical Research Unit at Amarillo. A special appreciation goes to Candace A. Myers, PhD for her invaluable guidance through all stages of editorial work.

Tetyana L. Vasylyeva, MD, PhD, DSc

Steps of Ideas Turnover

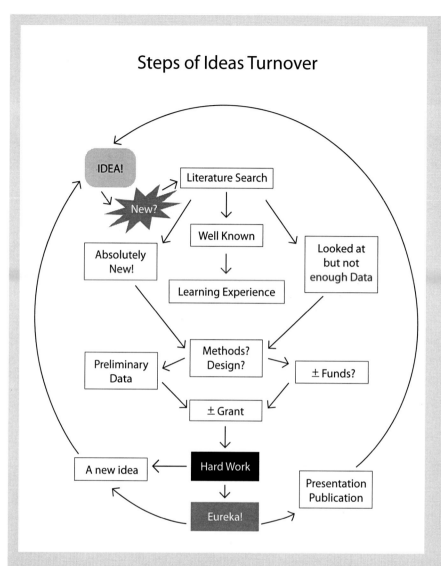

Figure 1.1. Roadmap of Research

1 | How to Address a Research Question

Matt Jeremiah T. Chua, MD

Christopher Giuliano, PharmD

Pradeep K. Selvaraj, MD, PhD

Mankind's curiosity and resiliency has driven civilization towards advancement throughout the course of history. Even before the advent of written language, prehistoric man was able to pass knowledge from generation to generation through oral traditions. Our ancestors were able to domesticate animals, develop agriculture, and acquire astronomical knowledge (Hamilton, 2009; Hillman, Hedges, Moore, Colledge, & Pettit, 2001; Ruggles, 2005). Aristotle introduced the law of logic using observation to explain different phenomena. This knowledge has led to the concept of deductive reasoning that we have today (Western Culture Global, 2009). The development of the *scientific method* follows the laws of logic. To be termed *scientific*, a method of inquiry must be observable, empirical, and measurable. Evidence must also be subject to specific principles of reasoning.

We practice today in an era of evidence-based medicine, in which we use the best available evidence, gathered using the *scientific method*, to apply to clinical practice and decision-making. Logic and reason are no longer enough. The requirement for evidence has led to a paradigm shift in the practice of medicine. For example, the use of beta-blockers was initially avoided in systolic heart failure patients due to their negative inotropic effects, which logically would worsen heart failure (Foody, Farrell, & Krumholz, 2002). Eventually, investigators studied the question and demonstrated a reduction in mortality with beta-blocker use in this population, and now their use in systolic heart failure is the standard of care.

Every good research project starts with a good research question. A research question is simply a question that a researcher develops to discover an answer. Our goal in this chapter is to give a practical guide to help researchers formulate research questions. Research questions usually stem from one's observations, previously published studies, and from discussions with colleagues (Hulley, Cummings, Browner, Grady, & Newman, 2007). The success of a research project starts with the research question. It is important to begin on solid footing because conducting research is a time-consuming, energy-draining, and expensive task. Here are some tips on originating good research questions:

1. **Master the Literature** - Conduct a thorough literature review on the subject of interest.

2. **Be Alert to New Ideas** - Conferences and forums are a good source of innovative ideas. New technologies generate new questions about familiar problems and create new paradigms.

3. **Be Creative** - Keep your imagination roaming and try to conceive research questions using new methods to address new or old problems.

4. **Choose a Mentor** - Research, as with other tasks, has a learning curve. An experienced mentor is of great value. The advice of an experienced researcher is one of the most valuable resources a new researcher can find.

There are many critical questions that you may need to address in formulating a research question. Do you have personal knowledge of or an interest in the field of study? Is there a need to reinvent the wheel? Or maybe just to improve the wheel? What is the impact of your proposed study? Do you want to try to reproduce a recent study with novel results and a small study population to further fortify the findings? This is quite commonly done. For example, bariatric surgery decreased hypertension in a cohort of pregnant patients in an Israeli study, and these findings were further confirmed in a larger study published in British Medical Journal (BMJ) (Bennett et al., 2010; Weintraub et al., 2008).

The two criteria that are commonly cited when developing a research question have the mnemonics PICOT and FINER.

PICOT Criteria (Table 1.1)

The PICOT criteria stands for **P**opulation, **I**ntervention, **C**omparison group, **O**utcome of interest, and **T**ime. These criteria are useful in the development of a *specific* research question (Haynes, Sackett, Guyatt, & Tugwell, 2006). The PICOT elements help to generate the framework of the research question and begin the process of protocol development. It is especially useful for formulating inclusion and exclusion criteria (Farrugia, Petrisor, Farrokhyar, & Bhandari, 2010).

Population – What specific population are you interested in studying?

A well-defined population with exacting inclusion and exclusion criteria will produce a focused and specific study with less bias, but may limit the applicability to a small group of patients. On the other hand, a broad population introduces more bias, but the applicability increases; therefore, it may be more practical in clinical practice (Farrugia et al., 2010).

Intervention – What is your intervention?

This includes the type of intervention, compliance, and safety concerns (Haynes et al., 2006). Who will administer the intervention should also be included here. For example, for surgical interventions, it is important to minimize bias by recruiting surgeons with similar expertise and experience; i.e., surgeons from referral centers with similar numbers of operations performed and similar track records.

Comparison – To what are you comparing your intervention?

Your treatment group can be compared to either a standard treatment group, a placebo group, or to varying components of treatment (e.g., same treatment but different doses).

Outcome of Interest – What do you intend to accomplish?

Time – what is the time frame of the study?

Now let us apply **PICOT:**

Among patients with symptomatic pulmonary hypertension (idiopathic, disease associated with connective-tissue disease, or due to repaired congenital systemic-to-pulmonary shunts) **[Population]** can sildenafil (20, 40, or 80 mg) **[Comparison]** orally three times daily **[Intervention]** for 12 weeks **[Time]** compared to placebo **[Comparison]** improve functional status? **[Outcome]**

Outcome must be a measurable variable. In this particular study, distance walked in six minutes, change in mean pulmonary artery pressure, World Health Organization (WHO) functional class, and the incidence of clinical worsening (defined as death, transplantation, hospitalization for pulmonary arterial hypertension, or initiation of additional therapies for pulmonary arterial hypertension, such as intravenous epoprostenol or oral bosentan) were used as outcome measurements (Galie et al., 2005).

Table 1.1. PICOT Criteria

Population	What is your specific population?
Intervention	What is your intervention?
Comparison	What are you comparing?
Outcome of Interest	What are you intending to accomplish?
Time	What is the time frame of the study?

FINER Criteria (Table 1.2; Hulley et al., 2007)

FINER stands for **F**easible, **I**nteresting, **N**ovel, **E**thical, and **R**elevant. This is a simple mnemonic to remember and use to assess the *character* of a good research question (Hulley et al., 2007).

Feasibility

Are you capable of carrying out the research project? Four components to consider when assessing feasibility are:

1. **Number of subjects**: This coincides with *Population* in the PICOT criteria. Are enough subjects available to enroll and can you limit the drop-out rate? You can use a preliminary statistical calculation of study power to estimate the needed sample size.

2. **Technical expertise**: Do the investigators possess the expertise to successfully conduct the research? This is where choosing a mentor may be important.

3. **Time and money**: Do you have the time to conduct the study and the money to pay for supplies, drugs, equipment, and help?

4. **Scope**: A good research question should be focused and well-defined. A good research question is never a *fishing expedition* or too broad with too many questions. Formulate a research question that has one primary target question. One or two sub-questions may be added, but be very careful not to lose focus (Panacek, 2007).

Interesting

The research question should be interesting to both the investigator and your intended audience (Durbin, 2004). If you do not find the research question interesting, you will probably lack the desire to put in the long hours to produce a quality project. This may lead to poor results. If the question is not interesting to your intended audience, your results may be difficult to get published, and if published may be ignored.

One way to develop an interesting research question is to find personal experiences in practice and translate these experiences into research questions. For example, you are tasked with researching different antiplatelet agents (clopidogrel versus dipyridamole/aspirin) to evaluate which agent would most effectively reduce a patient's risk of further ischemic strokes. After conducting a literature search, you find there are no high-quality data comparing the agents. This could lead you to pose the research question, "Is clopidogrel or dipyridamole/aspirin more effective at secondary prevention of ischemic strokes?" Practice-based research questions should be interesting to other clinicians in the same practice area.

Asking "why?" during your practice is an easy way to find interesting research questions, especially a new clinician (Lipowski, 2008). For example, you will inevitably ask yourself at some point within your training, "Why is this activity performed in this manner?" This question is often overlooked by senior clinicians who have been practicing for years, and this is a great way to find an area where more research needs to be done. Is performing procedure Y more effective than the old procedure X? Also, be on the lookout for irregular patterns that occur during practice. When rosiglitazone and pioglitazone were initially approved by the FDA, studies showed no differences in the incidence of congestive heart failure (CHF) between the medications and placebo (Hanefeld & Belcher, 2001; Lebovitz, Dole, Patwardhan, Rappaport, & Freed, 2001). Once on the market, a possible increase in CHF was noted in a series of case reports (Cheng & Fantus, 2004). The case series led to several trials, and eventually a meta-analysis showing an increased risk of developing CHF following long term (at least one year) treatment with rosiglitazone or pioglitazone (Lago, Singh, & Nesto, 2007). Staying alert to irregularities in practice will bring forth many interesting research questions.

Be sure to identify the audience that finds your data interesting and also what journal would be likely to publish your work. This will help to organize your thoughts, plan your trial design, and evaluate your outcomes. For example, if you plan on publishing in a journal focused on clinical practice, it would be prudent to conduct a clinical study. A laboratory-based trial might be perceived as irrelevant or uninteresting to the particular audience of that journal. A good way to ensure that a research question is interesting is to present the question to your peers. They can help refine your research question to reach its full potential.

Novel

What makes a research question novel? The simplest definition of a novel finding is discovering information that has never been previously reported. These findings may present in a variety of ways and are often an unanticipated secondary result of a different research question. For example, gabapentin was initially approved as a medication to treat seizures, but incidentally was found to be effective in treating neuropathic pain during early trials (Dougherty & Rhoney, 2001). This led to the research question, "Is gabapentin effective for treating neuropathic pain?" Due to this unanticipated observation and subsequent trials, gabapentin remains one of the most commonly used agents for the treatment of neuropathic pain, although it is rarely used to treat seizures (Rosner, Rubin, & Hestenbaum, 1996).

A common way to develop a novel research question is by identifying areas of need that have been communicated in the literature. These questions can be identified by looking in various research publications and identifying where the authors voiced a need for more research. Another approach to derive novel research questions is by examining different areas of clinical controversy. You will encounter these controversies on a daily basis, and there are plenty of opportunities to try to answer controversial questions. Be sure to carefully review the relevant literature to understand why the issue is controversial.

Ethical

To proceed in investigating your research question, your research protocol must be approved by an institutional review board (IRB). Research approval has been tightened over the years after cases of unethical research were reported (Blaumslag, 2005; Caldwell, Price, Schroeter, & Fletcher, 1973). Certain populations (including children, prisoners, pregnant women, and patients with impaired decision-making skills) require special approval from an IRB. If you wish to conduct research with special populations, contact your IRB for the details of processes that you will need to complete.

There are many considerations to ensure that your research project is ethical. One major goal of ethical research is to provide more possible benefit than possible risk to the research subjects. If the risk outweighs the benefit, then the trial should not be conducted. For example, some studies do not have a placebo group because it would be unethical to withhold treatment from patients if a treatment with known benefit exists. Prospective studies will have many more requirements than retrospective studies, which pose minimal risks to patients. Furthermore, prospective studies will need to recruit patients, which bring up many ethical issues. These issues range from providing monetary compensation without coercing people to participate, to selecting subjects in a fair manner. If you have any concerns about the ethics of your research, contact your IRB.

Relevance

When is a research question relevant? A good way to judge relevancy is to consider how the outcome of the research would improve scientific knowledge, influence clinical and health policy, and pave the way for future research directions. It is always important to think about the relevance before starting any research project. For example, if you want to study the exposure of oral bisphosphonates and risk of developing esophageal cancer, first think what is the importance of this study? How can the outcome influence the health of the general population? The plausible outcome of this study is either oral bisphosphonates increase or do not increase the risk of developing esophageal cancer. The relevance of this outcome will improve the scientific knowledge, influence the clinical practice by making physicians more vigilant of any signs of cancer, and pave the way for future research, such as improvising the molecular structure of bisphosphonates to decrease the cancer incidence.

Table 1.2. FINER Criteria

Feasible	Project manageable Adequate number of subjects Adequate technical expertise Affordable in time and money
Interesting	To yourself and intended audience
Novel	New findings Confirm or disprove previous findings
Ethical	Study that an institutional review board will approve
Relevant	To clinical practice and health policy To improve scientific knowledge To pave path for future research

Summary:

1. Any study must have a specific research question. The question must be interesting to both the authors and the intended readers. Tools to your advantage are being knowledgeable on the subject and open for ideas from experienced colleagues or mentors.

   - Ask a **specific question** for a specific answer.
     Vague question → Confusion
   - Question must be **Interesting** to you and your audience
   - Ask **novel** questions to improve scientific knowledge

2. There are two criteria that are commonly cited when developing a research question (FINER and PICOT criteria). These two criteria are useful in development of a good and specific research question.

   - **FINER:** Feasible, Interesting, Novel, Ethical and Relevant
   - **PICOT:** Population, Intervention, Comparison, Outcome of Interest, and Time.

3. The crucial step is to develop a good research protocol. It is important to have a hypothesis which is well defined. If the hypothesis is vague or unrealistic, the entire protocol will collapse. Always have a definite goal directed hypothesis.

> - Have a **Goal directed hypothesis**
> - Write a **hypothesis-driven protocol**

4. Once you established a hypothesis driven protocol, it is important to get recommendations or feedbacks from your mentor or colleague.

> - Review your **study protocol** with your **mentor** or experienced colleague

2 | Clinical Study Designs Overview

Tetyana L. Vasylyeva, MD, PhD, DSc

"Design is where science and art break even."
Robin Mathew

We all practice "evidence-based medicine," but to collect evidence, we need to have a clinical investigation. Clinical research is the cornerstone for evidence-based medical practice. Everything from large-scale studies that involve different centers (multicenter studies) in different cities or different countries, to retrospective chart reviews that focus on the medical records for a certain period of time at a single institution, or even a single case report can produce evidence.

The study design depends on the investigators' ideas, goals, and available resources. Let's consider what the options are:

Observational Studies

In a basic observational study, the investigator notes some new concept, paradigm, or issue in everyday practice, and compares it to what we already know. The greatest value of observational studies is that they gather the preliminary evidence to use to form future hypotheses for experimental studies. The path might originate from a single case report, a case-series, a cohort study, or a case-control study. Observational studies are also important to answer questions that would be unethical to assign, but are important to study when they occur. For instance, it would be unethical to expose a population to radiation, but observing the health ramifications of radiation exposure after the Chernobyl accident provided data on the impact of different levels of exposure on the health of people dwelling in surrounding areas.

Observational studies are useful when it is impossible to manipulate the independent variable. The data gathered and conclusions drawn can share practical experience among physicians and create a more general picture of how the medically important issue might be managed. A lot of knowledge about disease etiology has come from observational studies. A fascinating example of an observational study which led to a great discovery is the discovery of penicillin. In 1928 the biologist Alexander Fleming was working on the properties of *staphylococci* when he noted that one of the culture plates was contaminated by mold. The area around the mold colony was translucent, which made the researcher think of lysis. Fleming repeated the experiment using different bacteria and different types of mold and drew conclusions regarding the bactericidal properties of mold and the sensitivities of bacteria, which lead to the discovery of penicillin. It took more than ten years for biochemists to develop a stable, purified form of penicillin that could be used in the general population. In his Nobel Lecture, Alexander Fleming stated, "…I might have claimed that I had come to the conclusion, as a result of serious study of the literature and deep thought that valuable antibacterial substances were made by molds and that I set out to investigate the problem. That would have been untrue, and I preferred to tell the truth that penicillin started as a chance observation. My only merit is that I did not neglect the observation and that I pursued the subject as a bacteriologist" (Fleming, 1945).

Risk factors or exposures are often the independent variables that might lead to consequences, such as a disorder or disease – the dependent variable. Observational studies have limitations and bias. The investigator is a passive observer, who does not control allocation or assignment of factors under investigation. The combination of factors is self-selected by the subjects, and large confounding biases might occur. The symmetry of unknown confounders cannot be controlled.

Observational studies can be descriptive (case report, case series, descriptive epidemiology) or analytical (case-control studies and cohort studies).

Case Report

The case report is the most frequent research design conducted by students, residents, and fellows. When an unusual situation occurs during clinical practice, the observer describes the manifestations, clinical course, and prognosis of a single case. Although single case reports provide little empirical evidence to clinicians, they might be a good start to study a clinical condition. Many diseases have been named after the physicians who described them for the first time. For example, Down syndrome was first described by J. L. H. Down in 1866 (Down, 1866). Walker-Warburg syndrome was first reported by A. E. Walker in 1942, and M. Warburg addressed its heterogeneity in 1971 (Walker, 1942; Warburg, 1971). Alport syndrome was described in the British Medical Journal by A. C. Alport in 1927 (Alport, 1927).

The list of unique case reports is long, but what is very important is the fact that the first description attracted other physicians' attention, more cases were reported, and case series were conducted that led to further investigation of causes and pathogenesis. Thus, we all now know that Down syndrome is caused by trisomy 21 (Lejeune, Gautier, & Turpin, 1959), and some of the clinical features were incorporated into the preliminary phenotypic maps of chromosome 21 developed by Korenberg (1993). This knowledge led to cloning a gene (RCAN1; 602917) from the Down syndrome critical region that is highly expressed in brain and heart. This suggested that it might be a candidate for involvement in the pathogenesis of Down syndrome mental retardation and/or cardiac defects (Fuentes et al., 1995). Further research by Canzonetta et al. (2008) concluded that gene DYRK1A (600855) mediated deregulation of REST (600571), a very early pathologic consequence of trisomy 21 with the potential to disturb the development of all embryonic lineages. This line of study warranted a closer look into its contribution to

Down syndrome pathology, and led to new rationales for therapeutic approaches (Canzonetta et al., 2008). There is strong reason to hope that in the 21st century the chromosome 21 disorder might find its cure.

The point we want to stress with case reports is to be attentive. When you see unusual features of a disease, document your observations thoroughly, collect laboratory results, and take photographs or other images (if appropriate). Then make your observations public for other physicians to consider. Don't be negligent, lazy, or too busy; your case report might open a broad avenue for future study and even a cure.

Case Series

The case series is one of the most common study designs in the medical literature. If similar cases are repeatedly observed in clinical practice, the topic might deserve researchers' attention. Groups of more than ten patients might be presented as a case series. A typical example of a case series study is a study conducted by Abbasi et al., where reports of 82 patients with hepatocellular carcinoma helped to describe the clinico-pathological and radiological profile of the disease (Abbasi, Butt, Bhutto, Gulzar, & Munir, 2010).

Case reports usually describe the manifestations, clinical course, and prognosis of a condition in an individual.

An example of a case series with multiple cases is our paper "One disease, multiple manifestations," where we described cases of Langerhans cell histiocytosis – a disease that can have many different clinical presentations and is challenging to diagnose (Selvan, Vasylyeva, Turner, & Regueira, 2008).

Case reports are a good source of "preliminarily data" and can be used to develop a hypothesis for investigation using stronger study designs. With case reports, a sample of cases can be chosen by a researcher and often measurable risk factors can be described, but case series design cannot provide an estimation of risk. Disadvantages of this type of study include its lack of comparisons between groups, insufficient sample size, and inappropriate sample selection (e.g., lack of randomization).

Another example of a case series was conducted in France, where researchers observed 18 patients with sarcoidosis who underwent renal transplantation (Aouizerate et al., 2010). The subjects were identified retrospectively in eight French renal transplantation departments. Patient medical charts, demographics, and the outcome of their renal transplantations were reviewed. These data helped to establish that renal transplantation may be carried out safely in transplant candidates with sarcoidosis.

Both case reports and case series can be referred to as *"descriptive studies"* because the studies only describe the observations that were made of an individual or group of individuals. Neither of these designs shows temporal relationships between events and outcomes. Case selection bias may exist and the studies may lack statistical validity.

Cross-Sectional (Prevalence) Study

Cross-sectional studies assess research subjects at one point in time. Disease and risk factors can be measured at the same time, and subjects can be categorized into two categories: having and not having the risk factor. Each of these categories can be subdivided with regard to the presence or absence of disease. Prevalence of disease in a group which has the risk factor *vs.* prevalence of disease in a group which does not have the risk factor can be compared. Such comparative analyses make cross-sectional studies superior to case series, where there is only a description of the disorder.

The advantages of cross-sectional studies are that they are relatively inexpensive and multiple risk factors can be analyzed at the same time. Risk factors and disease can be associated, but causality cannot be proven. These studies lack any information on the timing of exposure and its relationship to outcomes. The major limitation of prevalence studies is that patients who completely recovered or died soon after developing the disease are often missed.

An example of a cross-sectional study is the research which was conducted by Koh et al. in Singapore when they studied acceptance of medical students by patients from private and public family practices and specialist outpatient clinics (Koh et al., 2010). The study was designed to conduct an anonymous cross-sectional survey from March through October 2007 of Singaporean or permanent resident patients attending 76 private teaching family practices, nine public teaching family practices, and eight specialty clinics in a public teaching hospital. Researchers learned that parents of children were least comfortable with student examinations, while patients between 41 to 60 years old were the most comfortable. Females were less comfortable than males with medical students, and Chinese patients were the least comfortable about being interviewed or examined by medical students among the ethnic groups queried. The investigators also concluded that family practice settings offered medical students a more receptive learning environment than specialty clinics. Although the data do not address whether or not patients would become more receptive with time, they did provide information that might be useful for medical student educators.

In another cross-sectional study, Crompton et al. looked into racial disparities in motorcycle-related mortality, and analyzed data from the National Trauma Data Bank collected between 2002 and 2006 (Crompton et al., 2010). The authors were surprised to discover that although black motorcyclists were more likely to use a helmet compared with their white counterparts, Black motorcyclists appeared more likely to die after a motor collision. This study led to further exploration of health disparities between racial and ethnic groups.

Ecologic (Aggregate) Study

The ecological study design is very useful when aggregate data on risk factors, including environmental factors and disease prevalence from different population groups are available. The comparison of groups might identify meaningful associations.

In addition to the usual biases that can arise in observational studies, ecologic studies suffer from several additional forms of bias unique to their design (Wakefield & Haneuse, 2008). One problem with this design is that it is impossible to judge the exposure at the level of the individual (Greenland & Morgenstern, 1989; Piantadosi, Byar, & Green, 1988). The only reliable way to characterize within-area variation in exposures and confounders, and hence control ecologic bias, is to collect and incorporate individual-level data

(Wakefield & Haneuse, 2008). Confounding variables could vary in different areas and be difficult to control (Bjork & Strömberg, 2005).

This is illustrated by a study conducted by Gadomski and colleagues. They were interested in whether economic stresses influenced child work hours on family farms because economic stresses are a frequently cited reason for using children to perform farm work (Gadomski, de Long, Burdick, & Jenkins, 2005). They explored the relationship between economic indicators and child agricultural work hours between January 2001 and October 2003. This ecologic study design compared trends in aggregate child work hours with national and regional economic indicators. Over 2,000 children living or working on 845 farms in central New York participated in the original study. The study design allowed Gadomski to conclude that increased child work hours were associated with periods of higher farm sector productivity, rather than with periods of economic stress.

Another typical example of an ecologic approach is a study designed by Coughlin and King (2010). Their goal was to determine the relationships between the ecologic measures of commuting time and use of public transportation in relation to breast and cervical cancer screening among women in U.S. metropolitan areas who participated in the 2004 and 2006 Behavioral Risk Factor Surveillance System surveys. The surveys showed that in metropolitan areas, transportation issues and other factors (e.g., Hispanic ethnicity, low income, and no physician visit in the past year) all played a role in whether a woman obtained cancer screening (Coughlin & King, 2010).

Although ecological studies are justifiably criticized for their multiple sources of bias, they remain a valuable instrument to address some important medical questions.

Case-Control Study

The case-control design is most often used in retrospective chart review studies. This type of study has the advantage of being inexpensive and can be conducted when it is convenient for the researcher. No patient's schedules, informed consent, or direct communications with patients are required.

Case-control is the best design to initially evaluate a condition's risk factors and can be especially useful to study rare diseases or medical conditions with long induction periods. In case-control studies, disease or other outcome variables in the population at risk are compared with a control group without the disease or other outcome, who were exposed to the same risk. Looking back in time, it is possible to analyze and compare the proportion of the cases and controls exposed and not exposed to the risk factor or condition under investigation. Overall, a case-control study provides better evidence for causation than a cross-sectional study. More than one risk factor for a disease or outcome can be examined simultaneously. Researchers often use odds ratio as an estimate of relative risk and logistic regression when analyzing case-control study data.

Unfortunately, bias is an important problem with case-control studies, too. A researcher does not have control over the past event, data are frequently missing, data accuracy is difficult to check, and there is no way to supplement the information that is found. It can be difficult for a researcher to remain objective in collecting exposure information. A tendency exists to look more carefully for cases than for controls. Objective measurements and "blinding/masking" group status is a good way to overcome such a bias. It would be useful if a person who collects data would be unaware of the subject's group status. Since case-control studies allow for the study of only one disease at a time, there is no way to calculate incidence, prevalence, or excess risk (the association between a specified risk factor and a specified outcome). Selection bias can be a problem. It is very important for the cases and controls to be sampled in a valid manner.

An interesting case-control study was published by Ravera et al. They studied the association between the use of commonly prescribed psychotropic medications and traffic accidents in the Netherlands (Ravera, van Rein, de Gier, & de Jong – van den Berg, 2011). A record-linkage database was used to perform a case-control study. The data came from three sources: pharmacy prescription data, police traffic accident data, and driving license data. Cases were defined as drivers who had a traffic accident that required medical assistance between 2000 and 2007. Controls were defined as adults who had a driving license and had no traffic accident during the study period.

Various variables, such as age, sex, medicine half-life, and alcohol use, were considered for the analysis and added validity to the study.

Cohort (Incidence, Longitudinal Study) Study

The cohort study is a type of observational study that can be retrospective (the event happened in the past), prospective (the subjects are tracked after the event, over a follow-up period), or a time series (a sequence of data points, typically measured at uniformly-timed successive time points). The group of subjects might have been, is, or will be exposed to some factor of interest, or has some condition that will be followed over time in order to study the consequences of the event. Usually, there is no control group, so risk cannot be studied. Not all subjects who were initially enrolled in the study will complete it. Subject loss can contribute to the cost of this type of study, but a cohort study can provide stronger evidence-based data than a case-control study. A panel study is a type of cohort study where a cross-section of the subjects is sampled at regular intervals.

An example of a longitudinal cohort study is the Framingham Heart Study (2011). The researchers recruited 5,209 men and women between the ages of 30-62 from the town of Framingham, MA, in 1948. The first round of extensive physical examinations and lifestyle interviews were analyzed for common patterns related to cardio-vascular disease. The subjects returned every two years for a detailed medical history, physical examination, and laboratory tests. In 1971, the study enrolled a second generation of 5,124 children (or spouses of the children) of the original participants (Framingham Heart Study, 2011). In April 2002, the study entered a new phase, the enrollment of a third generation of participants, the grandchildren of the original cohort. This incredible study has provided such valuable information that it is impossible to overestimate its input to the contemporary knowledge of risk factors related to cardiovascular disease. This study helped to build preventive strategies for high blood pressure, high blood cholesterol, smoking, obesity, diabetes, and physical inactivity.

A hybrid design is called a nested case-control or nested case-cohort study, where all cases and control subjects are extracted from a known cohort. Controls are disease- or outcome-free and selected randomly from the initial cohort, irrespective of outcome. A nested case-control study is a relatively economical way to search for a cause of an adverse health outcome. A population or cohort is identified and surveys or biological samples are collected (and frozen). The subjects are followed over time and additional surveys or specimens might be collected. Eventually, a small number of the cohort manifests the disease. A random group of the 'cases' and a random group of the 'controls' are selected from the population for inclusion in the nested case-control study. The samples from this relatively small group are thawed and analyzed. There are several advantages of this type of study. Surveys or interviews conducted at baseline are free of recall bias. Because specimens were collected long before the disease developed, any abnormalities in the results represent risk factors rather than the consequence of disease. Nested case-control studies are economical because only the samples from the nested subjects are thawed and analyzed.

An example of a nested case-control study is a recent study reported by Bradley et al., where the authors investigated the relationship between statin use and pancreatic cancer risk (Bradley, Hughes, Cantwell, & Murray, 2010) among subjects in a large research database. Cases developed a diagnosis of primary malignant neoplasia of the exocrine pancreas. Controls were matched with cases on general practice site, sex, and year of birth. The exposure of interest was use of statins. A total of 1,141 pancreatic cancer cases and 7,954 controls were identified. Authors found that neither dose nor duration of statin-use affected pancreatic cancer risk.

Meta-Analysis Study

Meta-analyses are classified as observational studies because they do not contain any experiments per se, but rather analyze previous analyses. Meta-analysis is useful when the number of subjects in the individual studies is not large enough to form significant conclusions. It is the integration of research through statistical analysis of the analyses of individual studies (Glass, 1976). The Cochrane Collaboration defines a meta-analysis as the use of statistical techniques in a systematic review to integrate the results of included studies (Cochrane Collaboration, 2011).

Meta-analysis is used to more precisely estimate the true "effect size" as opposed to a smaller "effect size" derived in a single study under a given single set of assumptions and conditions. Meta-analysis clearly has advantages over conventional narrative reviews and carries considerable promise as a tool in clinical research and health technology assessment (Egger, Smith, & Phillips, 1997). The meta-analyst must define the review's purpose and carefully identify appropriately similar studies. A weakness of the method is that sources of bias are not controlled. We would advise investigators to get a thorough statistician's review of the original studies before applying this method.

Chen et al. used meta-analysis to analyze clinical manifestations, diagnostic examinations, and methods of management of duplication cyst of the duodenum (Chen et al., 2010). The researchers reviewed related articles published from 1999 to 2009 on *PubMed* and found 38 citations in the literature that provided adequate descriptions of 47 cases of duodenal duplication cysts. Meta-analysis allowed them to determine that the most common symptom in duodenal duplication cysts is abdominal pain, with or without nausea or vomiting, and the most common complication is pancreatitis.

With a meta-analysis, Liu et al. answered a question about whether dietary fat was associated with an increased risk of colorectal cancer (Liu et al., 2010). In order to reach their research goal, the authors retrieved published literature from *Medline*, *Embase*, and *CNKI* (China Knowledge Resource Integrated Database) databases updated to May, 2009. Overall, 13 prospective cohort studies with 3,635 cases and 459,910 participants were included. They surprisingly found that dietary fat was not associated with an increased risk of colorectal cancer, in contrast with experimental animal findings.

Experimental Studies

Experimental studies provide the strongest evidence-based results if the studies are well-designed and bias is minimized. Investigators can control some bias by using random assignment to the study groups. Experimental studies are analytic. They are also prospective. A researcher must design it in advance to target a specific issue of interest. Thus, Rubin and McDonnell decided to determine the effect of a year-long, multifaceted diabetes curriculum on the knowledge of internal medicine residents (Rubin & McDonnell, 2010). In this controlled, prospective study, diabetes knowledge assessments were performed with a published questionnaire to measure baseline knowledge (PGY-1), determine change in knowledge at one year, and to compare resident knowledge with attending physicians' knowledge (control). They found that traditional educational methods may not be adequate and improved education strategies are needed for trainees to provide optimal diabetes care.

In experimental studies, researchers establish a certain goal (knowledge of diabetes) and choose the study groups (PGY-1) residents (an experimental group) and their faculty (a control group), and then follow them over the period of study (one year) to determine a result. The study is a good example of a prospective experimental study and might have the added benefit of teaching the students and residents about prospective study design.

Clinical trials can be referred to as treatment trials, prevention trials, diagnostic trials, screening trials, and quality of life trials. The study might be sub-divided as "superiority trials," in which the goal is to demonstrate that one treatment is more effective than another. Non-inferiority trials are designed to demonstrate that a treatment is not appreciably worse than another treatment, and an "equivalence trial" demonstrates that one treatment is as effective as another.

Randomized Controlled Clinical Trials

The randomized controlled study is the gold standard to generate evidence-based information in the clinical setting. Subjects are required to meet certain inclusion criteria and should not meet any exclusion criteria in order to be eligible to participate in the study. The eligibility criteria depend on the study's focus and goal. Usually, individuals who consented to participate in the study will be randomly assigned to two or more treatment groups. All participants will be followed over a period of time sufficient to draw a conclusion about the efficacy of the intervention.

You can easily locate examples of randomized controlled studies in *PubMed*. In general, an investigator decides to determine if an intervention is better than no treatment. In this case, the 'control' would be a placebo made to look like the pill being tested. In other studies, you might compare standard treatment to a new drug and determine if the new treatment is more effective than the old treatment or if it possesses some additional beneficial feature. In that case, the reference or control is the standard treatment.

The study can be open-label or single-, double-, or triple-blinded. In an open-label study, both the researchers and the subjects know which treatment the subjects are receiving. Blind studies are designed to prevent possible conscious or unconscious bias by withholding the actual treatment choice from the subjects and/or researchers. Such biases might relate to the placebo effect, observer bias, or conscious deception. Blinding can be imposed on researchers, technicians, subjects, funders, or any combination of study participants. In single blind trials, the subjects do not know whether they are getting drug X or drug Y, but the researcher is aware of the subjects' group assignments. With double-blind studies, an attempt to eliminate subjective bias on the part of both subjects and the healthcare providers is made by making some third party (often a pharmacist) responsible for group assignment. The doctors and subjects are all in the dark about the distribution of treatments until the code is broken at the end of the study. A triple-blind study is a double-blind study in which the identities of those enrolled in the study and control groups and/or the details about the nature of the interventions (experimental medications) are withheld from the statistician who conducts the analysis of the data.

Randomized controlled clinical trials are usually conducted with parallel groups over the same period of time to justify an effect (see also Chapter 5: Clinical Trials: Design and Monitoring).

Randomized Cross-Over Studies

Randomized cross-over clinical trials are often used to study treatments for chronic conditions. The advantage of this study design is that the same patients are exposed to both types of treatments, usually with a washout period in between. Although this design seems very attractive, bias remains an issue. The major concern is a time-effect relationship where the effect from the first treatment may carry-over for the second course of therapy (see also Chapter 5: Clinical Trials: Design and Monitoring).

A cross-over study design can be applied not only to medicine-related clinical trials, but also to address many other clinical tasks. For example, Van Eaton and colleagues employed a cross-over study design to answer the question, "Is a computerized rounding and sign-out system, designed to reduce resident duty hours, safe for the patients?" (Van Eaton et al., 2010). This 14-week, randomized, cross-over study involved 14 inpatient resident teams (six general surgery, eight internal medicine) at two hospitals. The authors measured resident-reported deviations in expected care, medical errors, and institutionally-reported adverse drug events. They found that the computerized system improved continuity and enhanced resident efficiency without weakening systemic defenses against error or jeopardizing patient safety.

Quasi-Randomized Trials

A trial using a quasi-random method of allocating participants is not truly random. In this design, allocation is determined by date of birth, day of the week, medical record number, month of the year, or some other unrelated criteria. There is a risk of increased selection bias in quasi-random trials where allocation is not adequately concealed compared with true randomized controlled trials.

A Before-After Study

This study design is used in many clinical studies to evaluate the impact of treatments or interventions. It has been used frequently in trauma-related studies. A before-after study measures disease issues at two (or more) time points, before the initiation of an intervention or treatment and at like intervals after the intervention. The goal of the design is to determine if there was a change over time. In theory, the change is attributed to the intervention. In the majority of studies, the time points are six and 12 months before and the same intervals after treatment. The major reason for the popularity of the before-after study design is the low cost, convenience, and simplicity in conducting the studies. It is useful in addressing the ethical issues that may come up with randomized studies or prospective cohort designs.

This study design does not have an external control. The comparison is done to the same group, but at the different time points. The presumption is that the intervention had a significant impact on the disease. Without a control group, it is difficult to establish the cause and effect relationship between the exposure and the effect. People might just change over time, such as a child involved in an experiment might grow over time and became a better learner. Before-after studies might be influenced by the statistical phenomenon of "regression to the mean" (left to themselves, things tend to return to normal).

Morrow wanted to improve rates of seatbelt use in young school children and their parents. He introduced and evaluated curricular interventions in a before-after trial over a 15-week period at a public school for pre-kindergarten through second grade (ages four to eight years) in Yonkers, NY. All of the 422 students at the school were included and finished the study. A sequential group of parent drivers were also evaluated, although they were not subject to an active intervention (Morrow, 1989). As a result of the intervention, belt use among students increased from 46% to 66%, and was re-measured one month later at 63%. Use of belts by parents improved from 47% to 61% (P < 0.01), and remained at 62% at the one-month follow-up.

Focus Groups

A description of study designs would not be complete without mention of focus groups. Focus groups perform qualitative analysis, mostly in psychology or other social group-related research. These studies usually involve a group of people who were asked about their perceptions, opinions, beliefs, and attitudes toward certain topics. Depending on the goal of the study, there are different types of focus groups (two-way focus groups, dual moderator focus groups, dueling moderator focus groups, and others). As with any other research design, it has its place and its drawbacks. One disadvantage of a focus group study is that the researcher has less control over a group than over a one-on-one interview. The data are tough to analyze because the conversation is in reaction to the comments of other group members, and the number of members of a focus group is not large enough to be a representative sample of a population.

An example of an application of focused group study can be found in a recent paper of Grace and Higgs. They used this design to study integrative medicine in an emerging model of healthcare (Grace & Higgs, 2010).

Another example is the work of Harman et al. when the authors described barriers to charting identified by physiotherapists working in private practice (Harman, Bassett, Fenety, & Hoens, 2009). They invited physiotherapists to focus group interviews to discuss the results of a comprehensive chart audit. Sixty-nine physiotherapists responded and were assigned to nine focus groups. The interviews were tape-recorded (Kim, Zakharkin, & Allison, 2010). Analysis of the data led to conclusions and suggestions about ways to improve the quality of documentation.

Translational Research

Although this book is dedicated to clinical research, it would be incomplete without some mention of translational research. A new era opened with the Human Genome Project that has resulted in significant advances in the understanding of the molecular mechanisms of complex disorders, including cancer, heart disease, and metabolic diseases (Kim et al., 2010). Gene-related clinical projects are the most prominent examples of translational research. Gene expression profiling, when used properly, offers the potential for the development of clinically-relevant biomarkers. Gene expression profile analysis is frequently controversial because it often lacks reproducibility, and claims of effective dissemination into translational medicine have, in some cases, been unjustified. In the last decade, a large number of methodological and technical solutions have been offered to overcome the challenges. DNA microarrays are widely used tools in biomedical research and fertile testing grounds for novel statistical methodologies. The studies require some specific approaches and designs, which are outside the scope of this chapter, but might be found in the following references (Baliga, 2008; Gilad, Rifkin, & Pritchard, 2008; Manolio & Collins, 2009).

An example of a translational study can be found in an article published by Van de Vijver et al. in the *New England Journal of Medicine*. They analyzed 295 patients with breast cancer and assessed a gene-expression signature as a predictor of survival (Van de Vijver et al., 2002).

Another example of translational research is a study by Sims, Willberg, and Klenerman. The authors designed a fluorescently-labeled tetrameric MHC-peptide complex to use to understand natural host defense, as well as vaccine design and assessment (Sims, Willberg, & Klenerman, 2010).

Choosing a Study Design

The selection of an appropriate study design hinges on the question of how to get the most valuable results. Many factors must be taken into account when making a decision about the study design. The most important factor to consider is the goal the researcher is trying to achieve by conducting the study. We described only the most widely used approaches, but most study designs can be modified to achieve the goal with no harm to the patients, minimal risk, and the highest yield of results. Bias should be minimized, and available resources and the number of available subjects must be considered.

Be creative with the design of the study! Many institutions in the U.S. now have dedicated Clinical Research Units, where experienced specialists help researchers choose the best possible design for a specific study.

3 | The Institutional Review Board (IRB) and Health Insurance Portability and Accountability Act (HIPAA) Regulations

Brian C. Weis, MD, PhD

Introduction

The "I" in "IRB" has been postulated to stand for a number of adjectives: "Irritating," "Impossible," "Irreproachable," etc. Though often maligned, the IRB, or Institutional Review Board, is a necessary entity at any institution where research on human subjects is performed. In order for a researcher to implement a protocol that involves humans as research participants, he or she must have approval from the IRB to assure that the well-being and safety of the subjects has been appropriately addressed in the research design. Thus, investigators must be familiar with the role of the IRB, the federal regulations enforced by the IRB, and the requirements necessary for successful approval of a research protocol by the board. The objectives of this chapter are to:

1. Provide a brief history of the IRB.

2. Describe the membership and function of the IRB.

3. Discuss the dialogue between the IRB and a research investigator conducting human subject research.

4. Provide practical recommendations for researchers who will interact with the IRB during the course of their research investigations.

5. Discuss: Health Insurance Portability and Accountability Act

The History of the Institutional Review Board

There was very little oversight concerning the safety of human research subjects until the late 1940s. The atrocities carried out by Nazi scientists on Jewish prisoners that were revealed during the Nuremberg trials following World War II led to the Nuremberg Code, the first declaration of the fundamental principles that should guide research on humans. The Code stated that human research subjects had the right to voluntary and informed consent, a favorable risk/benefit analysis, and the right to withdraw from the protocol without penalty. These tenets would become the cornerstones of regulations overseeing human subject research in the future.

In 1973, Senator Edward Kennedy convened a congressional panel to hear concerns raised by the public about the ethics of several human research studies. First, the Willowbrook Hepatitis Study in the 1950s used mentally handicapped children in a state institution to study the transmission of a hepatitis virus. In this study, otherwise healthy children were intentionally infected with the hepatitis virus by being fed food containing fecal matter from children with active hepatitis. In a second study in the 1960s, Stanley Milgram performed a study on the tendency of humans to follow authority despite apparent adverse consequences. Subjects in this study were encouraged to electrically shock another individual, a "learner," who was being asked to recall a set of numbers, but who would be punished for a mistake. Unbeknownst to the subjects, the shocks were not real, but the expressions of pain by the "learner" appeared to be real. Despite knowing that some of the shocks were achieving levels known to cause severe harm, many of the subjects would continue to provide shocks for the "learner's" mistakes at the encouragement of the research personnel. When many of these subjects were told that the research was really to see how people followed the instructions of authority figures despite being led to do harm to others, they suffered psychological trauma and depression because of their own inability to resist what they knew to be improper guidance by an authority figure. Third, the Tuskegee Syphilis Study conducted from 1932 to 1972 involved largely uneducated, African-American share-croppers in Tuskegee, Mississippi, who had contracted syphilis. The study was intended to document the natural history of the disease. However, when penicillin became available as an effective treatment for this destructive infectious disease, the decision was made to withhold the cure from a population of the study participants in order to fulfill the initial objectives of the study. The fact that this study was directed by the federal government heightened concerns of the public as to what ethical considerations by federal funding agencies were being given to studies involving human subjects and, particularly, vulnerable populations.

The hearings in 1973 led to passage of the National Research Act by Congress in 1974. This act initiated the creation of the Institutional Review Board system and proposed the original policies and procedures that an IRB must follow when reviewing a research study. The original regulations would be codified in 1981 by the Department of Health and Human Services (DHHS) as Title 45, part 46 of the Code of Federal Regulations. These DHHS regulations now called the Common Rule are common to most federal agencies, excluding the Food and Drug Administration that has its own codes for research involving humans. The National Research Act also created a special committee known as the National Commission for Protection of Human Subjects of Biomedical and Behavioral Research (National Commission). This body issued the Belmont Report in 1978, which now serves as the ethical foundation for all research involving human subjects.

The Belmont Report

The Belmont Report was a major milestone in the regulation of human research by laying out the ethical principles that guide IRBs in the review of research protocols. The first principle is respect for humans. Under this tenet, all humans are seen as **autonomous** agents who have the right to be fully informed, make completely voluntary decisions on participation in research, and be assured protection of privacy and confidentiality. Understandably, there are individuals who cannot make fully informed and voluntary decisions due to mental or physical impairments. Others may have situational constraints on their freedom, such as persons in prisons or state institutions. Both groups would fall under the title of "vulnerable populations." The Belmont Report affords extra protection to vulnerable populations under this principle. The second principle is **beneficence**. This holds that in any research project where humans are subjects, the design must maximize potential benefits and minimize risks. The third principle is **justice**. This states that the potential risks of the research must be borne equally by the members of society likely to benefit from the results of the investigation. Members of the IRB are required to have thoroughly read the Belmont Report and be competent in applying its basic tenets to the research protocols brought before the board.

The Make-Up of the IRB

The IRB is meant to be a committee composed of individuals who represent a cross-section of the community in which the research is performed. The primary responsibility of this board is to protect the rights and well-being of human research participants. The DHHS regulations state that the IRB should consist of at least five members. Among the members, the committee must have at least one scientist, one nonscientist, and one person who is not directly affiliated with the research institution. Once these requirements are met, the IRB must then contain members of sufficient expertise to reasonably review the protocols that are submitted to the Board. For most IRBs, other members consist of physicians, pharmacists, statisticians, students, and representative members of the community that are outside the medical field. Frequently, one of the community members is an attorney; otherwise, legal counsel is normally available on a consultation basis. A given institution may have one or more individual IRBs, depending upon the volume of protocols generated for review. IRBs meet no fewer than one time per month, some more frequently than that. A meeting can only be called to order if a majority (greater than 50%) of the board's members are present.

Leadership for the IRB comes in the form of the IRB chairperson and the IRB administrator. While most positions on the committee are voluntary, the chairperson and administrator are normally compensated for their time by their institution. The chairperson's job is to run the meetings, mediate discussion amongst the members, and oversee the communications with the institution's research investigators. The IRB administrator is normally the person of contact for the researchers. The administrator distributes the review responsibilities, prepares the meeting agenda, transcribes the minutes, and finalizes all documents to be sent to investigators for protocols under review. Unlike in previous times when all of the research materials were on paper, many IRBs today use electronic systems through which the research protocol documents are submitted and reviewed. Not only does this minimize the use of paper, it hastens the committee meetings by allowing for more rapid access and review of the research materials.

Any protocol that uses human subjects must be submitted to and approved by the IRB. The initial submission will be categorized in one of three ways: exempt from IRB review, eligible for expedited review, or requiring full board review. Normally, these designations are decided upon by the IRB administrator or IRB chair. An exempt protocol must meet at least one of several criteria established by the DHHS:

1. The research is conducted in an established or commonly accepted educational setting and involves normal educational practices.

2. The research involves the use of educational tests, survey procedures, interview procedures, or observations of public behavior that do not permit identification of individuals or place the individuals at risk of liability or damage to their financial status or reputation.

3. The research involves the collection or study of existing data, documents, records, pathological specimens, or diagnostic specimens, if these sources are publicly available.

4. The research projects are designed and conducted to study, evaluate, or otherwise examine public benefit or service

programs or the means in which services are obtained or reimbursed under those programs.

5. The research is on taste and food quality evaluation and consumer acceptance studies.

Any protocol that meets one or more of these criteria can be considered exempt from IRB review. However, the IRB reserves the right to oversee such research if significant risk to study participants exists.

An expedited review is normally conducted by the IRB chair or other member designated by the IRB leadership. The DHHS and FDA regulations specify that a protocol can undergo expedited review if the activities present no more than minimal risk or the submission is for minor changes to a previously approved protocol during the approved period. The definition of "minimal risk" is that the probability and magnitude of harm or discomfort anticipated in the research are no greater than the risk ordinarily encountered in daily life or during the performance of routine physical or psychological examinations or tests. All protocols that receive expedited review must meet the standards of sound research design, including appropriate use of methodology and statistics, proper informed consent when necessary, data monitoring, and maintenance of confidentiality and privacy of research subjects. Protocols cannot be disapproved if under expedited review. If a protocol is questionable, it will be sent for a full board review.

Any protocol that proposes research involving greater than minimal risk to the human subjects must go before a full-board review. In this setting, the protocol is initially reviewed by a primary and secondary reviewer. The primary reviewer is commonly a person with scientific or clinical background, and the secondary reviewer is frequently a community member. The objective of the review is to determine that the design of the study has minimized risk and maximized benefit for the human research. The reviewers' job is to examine all study documents, including the informed consent form, to assure that the study subject is made fully aware of the details of the study and the risk associated with participation in the research. It is not unusual for the protocol to be returned to the investigator after the initial review with a list of "stipulations" for approval that are requested by the IRB. The stipulations can range from required modifications to the protocol or informed consent form to requests for clarification or supporting documentation on aspects of the research protocol. Whether or not the investigator completely agrees with the opinion of the IRB, the fastest way to obtain approval is for the researchers to comply with the stipulations and resubmit the protocol to the IRB. Most protocols will be approved either during the next board meeting or through an expedited process once the stipulations have been met.

Continued Dialogue with the IRB

Once an investigator's protocol has received approval on its initial review, the researcher will be given permission to implement his or her study by means of a letter from the IRB. This letter begins a dialogue process between the researchers and the IRB that will continue throughout the duration of the research project. Investigators will be expected to keep the IRB updated on any changes or developments with their protocols. Further submissions to the IRB can include one or more of the following:

1. Continuing Reviews (CR) – The investigator will be requested to provide scheduled periodic updates that include information on recruitment of participants to the study, safety reports or updates from sponsoring organizations, and any adverse events or protocol deviations that have occurred. The CR is normally submitted at no fewer than an annual frequency. If the study has been closed to accrual of new subjects, then the CR will receive an expedited review as the researchers continue the project solely to follow patients or analyze data.

2. Protocol Deviations – If a subject in the protocol has received treatment that deviated from the research protocol, a protocol deviation form must be submitted to the IRB that details the event and provides an explanation for the alteration. If the deviation was due to an oversight by the investigator, the report should also include an action plan on how such errors will be avoided by the investigators in the future. Any deviation that results in harm to a study subject will be taken

seriously by the IRB and could result in the IRB suspending enrollment in the study until a root-cause analysis can be performed and actions are taken to prevent any further deviations.

3. Protocol Amendment – Any change or modification to the protocol or informed consent must be submitted as an amendment to the IRB. Such changes can be as simple as the addition or subtraction of study personnel or as complicated as full revisions of the study protocol with associated changes to the informed consent. In situations where an amendment may alter the risk of the protocol, subjects who have already been enrolled may need to be consented again with the new informed consent form, so they are made fully aware of the change in risk.

4. Adverse Event – An adverse event is defined as any unpredicted outcome or harm that occurs to a subject on a protocol. This can include both events that are immediately related to the study protocol, such as a reaction to a study drug or procedure, as well as those that are completely unrelated, such as a study participant being hospitalized for an unrelated ailment. Even when the incident is clearly unrelated to the subject's study involvement, the researchers should submit their knowledge of the event to the IRB, so the IRB can monitor the well-being of the study participant.

5. Statement of Closure – Once the protocol has been completed, the research investigators should notify the IRB that the project is being closed to further activity. The IRB will end its oversight of the protocol at that time.

It is important that any of these reports to the IRB be submitted in a timely manner, namely, as soon as the investigator becomes aware of the reportable situation. The IRB does have the authority to suspend a study if the board feels that the investigators are deviating from the approved protocol or are not providing appropriate oversight to insure the safety of their study subjects. An open and honest discourse with the IRB is the investigator's best approach to prevent unwanted disciplinary actions by the board.

The Health Insurance Portability and Accountability Act

The Health Insurance Portability and Accountability Act (HIPAA), originally known at the Kasselbaum-Kennedy Act of 1996, was passed to make health insurance portable and to increase the accountability in Medicare billing. However, a section of this legislation deals with the storage and transmission of healthcare information. In support of this, the DHHS wrote two new regulations: the Standards for Privacy of Individually Identifiable Health Information (the Privacy Rule) and the Security Standards for the Protection of Electronic Protected Health Information (the Security Rule). These regulations were subsequently codified in 45 CFR 160-164. Both regulations assure that health information that can be traced back to a particular individual (protected health information or PHI) is strictly forbidden to be used for research or other purposes unless the individual provides his/her authorization. For the research investigator, this means that each study subject must sign an authorization for the disclosure of protected health information before the investigators can gather identifiable medical data on that individual.

The authorization for disclosure of protected health information must contain several key components. First, the form must state to whom the PHI will be disclosed. This includes not only the investigators performing the study, but also potential monitoring organizations, including funding groups, such as the National Institutes of Health (NIH), the IRB, and compliance regulators at the sponsoring institution. Second, the form must state what types of PHI about the study subject will be obtained and recorded by the investigators. These data can include everything from medical history to physical and laboratory examinations and radiologic studies. The subject must be fully informed as to what information concerning his/her health will be stored by the investigators for the research. Lastly, the HIPAA form must state that the subject can withdraw at any time from the study and prohibit further acquisition of protected health information on them. The subject does not have to be assured that the information that has already been gathered on them will not be used in the study analysis.

Certain studies, such as retrospective chart reviews, can gather medical information on subjects without gathering personal identifiers that link the medical information back to a particular individual. For example, a study on hypertension in a doctor's office could involve recording the blood pressure measurements of the first 100 patients without recording any other information that could identify to whom the blood pressure measurement belonged. In this case, a HIPAA waiver can be submitted to the IRB for the study stating that there is a minimal risk that any PHI will be disclosed for reasons of the protocol. This situation frequently coincides with a waiver of consent in studies that are deemed to be of minimal risk.

In all studies, the protection of health information concerning an individual is as important to the IRB as protection of the subject's personal well-being. The investigator must assure the IRB that all data and identifiable health information is stored in a manner that prevents unapproved access. For many investigators, this means assigning each subject a unique study number under which the PHI is filed. A list is then created that links the study number to an individual name, but this list must be stored in a location or manner such that only approved personnel can have access to this document. Most IRB applications will require a specific plan as to how the subject data will be stored and protected from unauthorized access.

Secrets to Working with the IRB

The IRB tends to be very busy; the volume of initial and continuing reviews, as well as the miscellaneous amendments and adverse event forms, can make the meetings long. Not infrequently, IRB members can become impatient and somewhat irritable. For this reason, it is of the utmost importance that an investigator avoid oversights in documentation that make the job of the IRB member more difficult. Nothing will kill a protocol in committee faster than improper completion of the required forms or inadequate provision of the research documents. With this in mind, I would make the following recommendations:

1. Be sure that all items on the submission checklist have been provided. This includes both the IRB submission form and

the protocol documents, including the consent form and the HIPAA authorization or waiver.

2. Be sure that grammar and spelling have been checked on all the documents.

3. When summarizing the project, use a brief and clear explanation of the research hypothesis and the design to be used to answer the research question. Remember, many of the members of the IRB are nonscientists, so simple terminology will work best.

4. Answer all questions on the IRB application honestly and completely. Check to make sure that the answers are consistent with the details of the study. Protocols can be returned without being voted upon simply for clarification of answers on the IRB application, even if the protocol itself is sound.

5. Make sure that the consent form is formatted properly and written at the suggested reading level (normally no higher than a 5th grade level). By far, consent form problems make up the majority of reasons for a protocol to be returned to the investigator without a committee vote.

6. Anticipate questions that the IRB may have with regard to safety concerns, and address them clearly in the consent form and protocol. Providing additional information from the medical literature can help give the IRB members perspective on the standard practice of a particular research technique.

If the IRB returns a protocol without approval, it is only natural for the investigator to become irritated and defensive. My recommendation is to avoid confronting the IRB. In these situations, the IRB will always win. An investigator will be best served by addressing the stipulations as best as possible and resubmitting the protocol without confrontation. Researchers who earn the reputation of being "difficult" by the IRB will only pay the price for this with all subsequent admissions. Investigators who demonstrate that they respect the system and can work within the rules will frequently be given the benefit of the doubt in future discussions by the IRB.

For young investigators, the IRB can provide valuable lessons in research design and implementation. Many larger health Sciences Centers will have a separate scientific review board that examines the merit and design of research protocols prior to review by the IRB. However, for the majority of smaller institutions, the IRB can serve both functions. Members of the IRB frequently have personal experience in conducting research studies. By simply reading the number of protocols that come through the review board, most of the IRB members become proficient in determining the quality and feasibility of research initiatives. Though the chief concern of the IRB is patient safety, the board will frequently focus on the use of resources, particularly if a protocol's design appears that it will not produce useful or relevant data. In other words, even if the research is safe, it is not worth doing unless there is some assurance that the research question that has been posed will be answered by the study design. Researchers should take advantage of the experience of the board and seriously consider the observations made by the members on any protocol reviewed.

Serving on an IRB can be an enriching experience for any investigator who wants to gain experience and insight into clinical research design. Though often seen as an obstacle to conducting research, the IRB can truly be a valuable resource at any institution where human research studies are conducted.

The ultimate resource for everything about the IRB is *Institutional Review Board: Management and Function* by Elizabeth A. Bankert, MA, and Robert J. Amdur, MD, (Bankert & Amdur, 2006).

4 | Informed Consent to Participate in Research

Kathy Thomas, RN, CIP

People are familiar with the procedure of signing documents that give their healthcare providers permission to provide and bill for service (Encyclopedia of Everyday Law, 2003). The goal of these forms is to ensure that patients have enough information about a procedure or treatment to decide if they agree with the proposed care. Informed consent for research participants is similar to informed consent for clinical care, but important additional criteria are required for research.

The distinction between informed consent for research versus informed consent for general practice begins with the physicians' justification for the intervention (Kluge, 2007). The purpose of research is to contribute to generalizable knowledge. The individual being approached to participate in the research activity is therefore a subject of interest. The study intervention is not primarily directed to an individual's well-being. This distinct difference must be acknowledged and addressed when obtaining a subject's consent to participate in research.

In private practice, a physician's intent is to provide healthcare with the anticipation of providing some benefit to the patient. The patient likewise expects the physician's activities to be directed toward their personal benefit. In most cases, the benefit of a research project intervention is unknown, and that is the reason for conducting the research. Subjects should be given an adequate opportunity to understand this difference in a setting that allows for confidentiality. Potential subjects should have the freedom to privately refuse to participate in the research.

When a patient agrees to participate in a research study, they become a subject and their personal and medical information (previously used to direct and pay for their medical care) may then be used as data. This distinction, patient versus subject, requires careful consideration on the part of the physician-researcher. This is especially true if the population to be studied is from a physician's private practice. In some clinic settings, the study personnel obtaining the consent are not associated with the provision of primary care. This is done to try to prevent the subject from assuming that participation in the research project is somehow related to their medical care and will also be directed toward their personal benefit.

When a medical research study recruits subjects from the general population, there may be less risk of confusion regarding benefit (Henderson et al., 2007). An example of this could include a pharmacokinetic study that administers a known drug to a healthy volunteer population and draws blood at pre-specified timed intervals to analyze for blood levels of the drug. The informed consent in such a project must clearly present the risk in conjunction with the known lack of benefit to the subject.

Informed consent is the ethical cornerstone of human research (Bankert & Amdur, 2006; Mascalzoni, Hicks, Pramstaller, & Wjst, 2008; Rosoff, 1981). Federal and State laws recognize that research subjects have inherent rights and research investigators have inherent duties. People have the right to determine what happens to their bodies, and doctors have a duty to provide sufficient information to ensure that each research subject can make a decision based on knowledge of his/her condition, the available options for treatment, known risks, and his/her prognosis.

Federal Regulations

Federal regulations establish basic protections for human subjects. State laws may provide additional provisions to be complied with, but they may not replace or take away from what is stated in federal regulations (Schwartz, 2001). The "Common Rule" is a reference term for the core of federal regulations that describes the protections of human subjects involved in research. Seventeen federal agencies and offices comply with these rulings, with the Office for Human Research Protections in the U. S. Department of Health and Human Services (2009) and the Food and Drug Administration (2011) heading the list. The regulations provide for heightened protections of certain vulnerable research subjects, such as pregnant women, fetuses, prisoners, and children.

The federal requirements characterize the environment, the information provided, the recipient, and the documentation for the process of informed consent for research participants (U.S. Department of Health and Human Services, 2009; Food and Drug Administration, 2011).

The Environment

When obtaining informed consent, the investigator should provide an environment that the potential subject will perceive as non-coercive, that will offer an unhurried opportunity to consider participation/non-participation in the study, and that demonstrates respect for the potential participant. A busy hallway would not be a proper setting to obtain informed consent. The information on the written consent form may be read to the subject or the legally authorized representative. The subject or their authorized representative must be allowed adequate opportunity for consideration prior to signing. This may require physicians to plan discussions to be held outside of busy clinic hours in a meeting place that can minimize interruptions.

The Information

The information on a research consent form must be provided in a language understandable to the recipient. This means that the text should be written at a fifth to eighth grade reading level. The subject will not be required to waive or appear to waive any legal rights, and the investigator will not be released or appear to be released from liability due to negligence. The same holds for the research sponsor, institution, or their employees. The document must include the following information:

- An explanation of the purpose of the research
- The anticipated length of time a participant would be expected to participate
- Reasonably foreseeable risks or discomforts
  - If appropriate, the effect on an embryo or fetus if the subject were to be or become pregnant
  - If appropriate, the fact that there may be unforeseeable risks
- Potential benefits to the participant (if any) or to others
- Appropriate alternative procedures or courses of treatment
- The extent to which confidentiality of records will be maintained
- Whether any compensation is provided
  - If appropriate, any additional costs to the subject that may result from participation in the research
- Whether medical treatment is provided in the event of an injury, and if so, what does this consist of, and where could further information be obtained, including who would be contacted in the event of an injury
- Who to contact for answers related to questions about the research
- Who to contact for answers related to questions about the participant's rights as a research subject
- A statement that participation is voluntary, refusal to participate will not result in a penalty or removal of care/benefits that would otherwise have been offered
- A statement that withdrawal from the research would not result in a penalty or removal of care/benefits that would otherwise have been offered

- As necessary, a description of the consequences of early withdrawal and the orderly way this can be performed
- If circumstances can be anticipated under which a subject's participation may be terminated by the investigator without regard to the subject's consent, this must also be stated
- A statement that any significant new findings developed during the course of the research which may relate to the subject's willingness to continue participation will be provided to the subject
- The approximate number of subjects expected to be involved in the study

Example: An adult patient presents to the clinic with flu-like symptoms. The patient has signed the institutional consent for treatment to allow any necessary samples or interventions to provide for their medical care. He/She has also completed a health assessment history (questionnaire) required by the clinic. A nasal swab will be taken as a part of the clinic routine to assist in determining their care.

An approved study is being conducted in this patient population that requires a second nasal swab for an additional laboratory test and the subject's cooperation in answering a brief research questionnaire. The subject will not receive the lab results from the nasal swab taken for research purposes or the cumulative results of all the participants who answered the questionnaire.

An informed consent form is required prior to any study intervention. Care must be taken to avoid confusion of clinical care with research participation. The physician investigator or a member of the research team would provide the patient with a brief description of the study, provide a copy of the written consent form, and allow the patient adequate time to read the information in private. The investigator or research team member would review the written information with any patients interested in participating, allow for questions, and obtain the necessary signatures. The swabs and questionnaire would follow. Considerations in planning this research project may include: what study team member will be responsible for the consent process (physician vs. study coordinator), space available to allow for a private research discussion in a busy clinic, and where research supplies will be maintained.

The Recipient

The consent must come from the subject or the subject's legally authorized representative (Bankert & Amdur, 2006; Texas Statutes, 2009). Adults are defined as persons 18 years of age or older or a person under 18 years of age who has had the disabilities of a minority removed (emancipated minor). Adults are generally presumed to be competent. Competence (capacity) includes the conceptual ability to understand the nature and implications of participation in a research study. Incapacitated means lacking the ability, based on reasonable medical judgment, to understand and appreciate the nature and consequences of a treatment decision, including the significant benefits and harms of, and reasonable alternatives to, any proposed treatment decision.

Children, adults with limited intelligence, and people with certain types of dementia are conceptually incompetent. Additionally, people with attention or memory dysfunctions who are unable to focus their attention on specific topics may be considered incompetent or lacking the capacity to offer consent.

A surrogate decision-maker (may also be known as a legally appointed guardian, legally authorized representative) is an adult with decision-making capacity, who is identified as the person who has authority to consent to medical treatment on behalf of an incapacitated patient in need of medical treatment. Legal documents can specify these individuals. In Texas, surrogate-decision makers are considered in the following order of priority:

1. Patient's spouse
2. Adult child of the patient who has the waiver and consent of all other qualified adult children of the patient to act as the sole decision-maker
3. A majority of the patient's reasonably-available adult children
4. The patient's parents

5. The individual clearly identified to act for the patient by the patient before the patient became incapacitated, the patient's nearest living relative, or a member of the clergy.

The medical treatment a surrogate consents to must be based on knowledge of what the patient would desire, if known. Surrogate decision-makers may not consent to voluntary inpatient mental health services, electro-convulsive treatment, or the appointment of another surrogate decision-maker. Disputes are resolved in court.

Texas, for example, does not have a specific statute addressing the conduct of human research. However, human research is referenced in several Texas statutes. Where specific research references are absent, the statutes that describe patient care may be substituted. Therefore, in Texas, the surrogate decision-maker can also consent for most research activities.

Children

Children are people who have not attained the legal age (age of majority) in the jurisdiction in which the research will be conducted. A child's biological or adoptive parent or an authorized guardian under applicable state or local law must consent on behalf of a child to take part in clinical research. The federal regulations very specifically outline the type of research that may involve children and the conditions that must be met.

The IRB will determine if the permission of one parent is sufficient for the proposed research. The project cannot involve greater than minimal risk, or it must present the possibility of direct benefit to the individual child-subject if the research involves greater than minimal risk. If the research involves greater than minimal risk and offers no prospect of direct benefit to individual subjects, but is likely to yield generalizable knowledge about the subject's disorder or condition, then permission must be solicited from both parents. Exceptions to obtaining both parents' permission include cases when one parent is deceased, unknown, incompetent, not reasonably available, or only one parent has legal responsibility for the care and custody of the child.

If the IRB determines a research protocol is designed for conditions or for a subject population for which parental/guardian permission is not a reasonable source to protect child-subjects (for example, neglected or abused children), the consent requirements may be waived, provided that an appropriate mechanism for protecting the children as subjects is substituted and the waiver is not inconsistent with other federal, state, or local law.

Assent of the Child

Provisions must be made to solicit the assent of the child. Assent is a child's affirmative agreement to participate in research. Mere failure to object should not be construed as assent. The determination for assent is made by the IRB and takes into account the age, maturity, and psychological state of the children involved in the research. If the intervention or procedure involved in the research holds a prospect of direct benefit that is important to the health or well-being of the child as a subject, and the intervention is available only in the context of the research, assent may be waived by the IRB.

The pregnant teenager is a complex area. It involves age – minor *vs.* adult or "age of minority" *vs.* "age of majority." It involves roles – parent vs child. Regulations address issues from both perspectives.

Wards of the State or any other Agency

In the case of children who are wards of the State or other agencies, permission by a guardian or *in loco parentis* is required. Additional permission is required from an advocate. An advocate is an adult who has the background and experience to act in, and agrees to act in, the best interests of the child for the duration of the child's participation in the research, and who is not associated in any way (except as advocate or member of the IRB) with the research, the investigator(s), or the guardian organization.

Example: A two-year-old has been diagnosed with acute leukemia. Verification of the specific type of leukemia for research purposes requires a bone marrow biopsy. The findings of the study could result in generalizable information about the child's disease. The project involves greater than minimal risk, so consent of both parents would be required. Special informed consent considerations will include the parent's emotional state and their ability to understand the research scope. Assent would not be required of a two-year-old, but generally children over the age of seven must agree to take part in the study, even if parental consent were obtained.

Pregnant Women, *In Vitro* Fertilization, and/or Fetuses

When research involves pregnant women, *in vitro* fertilization, and/or fetuses, additional specific federal stipulations apply.

1. If the research holds out the prospect of direct benefit to the pregnant woman, the prospect of a direct benefit both to the pregnant woman and the fetus, or no prospect of benefit for the woman nor the fetus when risk to the fetus is not greater than minimal and the purpose of the research is the development of important biomedical knowledge that cannot be obtained by any other means, the consent of the adult pregnant female is obtained in accord with the informed consent provisions previously stated.

2. If the research holds out the prospect of direct benefit solely to the fetus, then the consent of the pregnant woman and the father is obtained in accord with the informed consent provisions previously stated. Exceptions for obtaining the father's consent include: unavailability, incompetence, temporary incapacity, or the pregnancy resulted from rape or incest.

3. Each individual providing consent is fully informed regarding the reasonably foreseeable impact of the research on the fetus or neonate.

4. For pregnant children (defined as people who have not attained legal age in the jurisdiction in which the research is conducted), assent, and permission of the pregnant child's parent or legal guardian is obtained.

No inducements (monetary or otherwise) will be offered to terminate a pregnancy. Researchers will have no part in decisions regarding the timing, method, or procedures used to terminate a pregnancy or determine the viability of a neonate.

Example: An investigator is interested in assessing the prevalence of methicillin-resistant *Staphylococcus aureus* (MRSA) in pregnant women just prior to delivery. The study will require a vaginal swab. The results will not be shared with study participants. The test will not affect the fetus. There is no benefit to the study participant or the fetus. In this case, only the consent of the mother would be sought.

After admission for delivery, multiple vaginal exams are anticipated prior to delivery. The risk posed by swabbing is less than minimal risk for both the mother and fetus. An informed consent form is required prior to the study intervention. Special considerations in this case include the age of the mother (females less than 18 years old require parental consent) and the emotionally-charged environment during the delivery period. Depending upon the mother's proximity to delivery and other variables, a discussion about a research study during labor may be inappropriate or unwelcome. The investigator might consider discussing the study during a prenatal clinic visit and sending the consent form with the patient to consider prior to labor and delivery.

Prisoners

A prisoner is any individual involuntarily confined or detained in a penal institution. The definition includes detainment pending arraignment, trial, or sentencing. The federal regulations very specifically outline the type of research to be allowed, the conditions to be met, and the criteria for subject selection. The only topics that can be researched using prisoner participants are:

1. Study of criminal behavior and of the possible causes, effects, and processes of incarceration that presents no more than minimal risk and no more than inconvenience to the subjects.

2. Study of prisons as institutional structures or of prisoners as incarcerated persons that presents no more than minimal risk and no more than inconvenience to the subjects.

3. Research on conditions particularly affecting prisoners as a class (for example, vaccine trials and other research on hepatitis which is much more prevalent in prisons than elsewhere, and research on social and psychological problems, such as alcoholism, drug addiction, and sexual assaults).

4. Research on practices, both innovative and accepted, which have the intent and reasonable probability of improving the health or well-being of the prisoner subjects. In studies that require the assignment of prisoners to control groups that may not benefit from the research, additional permissions may be necessary.

In addition to the normally required components, informed consent among prisoners must include a clear explanation that research participation will not affect parole. If follow-up examinations or care could be required, adequate provision must be made for the varying lengths of individual prisoner's sentences and considerations for study participation.

Documentation

Unless otherwise allowed by the IRB, informed consent and assent shall be documented by the use of a written consent form that has been approved by the IRB and signed by the subject or the subject's legally-authorized representative. Usually, the consent form includes the information described above. In some cases, a short form stating the elements of informed consent are presented orally and a written summary of what is to be said to the subject or representative is submitted for IRB approval. In this case, a witness to the presentation signs both a copy of the short form and a copy of the written summary. The person obtaining the consent signs a copy of the summary. Copies of the short form and the written summary are provided to the subject or legal representative.

If the only record linking the subject and the research would be the consent document, and a breach of confidentiality could result in harm to the subject, the IRB may waive the consent. Documentation may also be waived if the research presents minimal risk of harm and involves no procedures that would require consent outside the context of research.

Example: A research project involves recruitment of abused adult women to complete a questionnaire regarding access to resources. The assessment is a one-time questionnaire. The results will be compiled, and the only record linking the subject to the research would be the consent document. Informed consent considerations may be associated with the recruitment technique and include: 1) oral presentation of the study by research personnel to a group of women at a women's shelter to allow questions to be answered, 2) distribution of the questionnaire with instructions not to write their names on the questionnaire, and 3) instructions to place the completed questionnaire in a designated sealed box in the back of the room for pick-up by the research personnel at a later time. In this case, an IRB might waive documentation of consent because minimal risk of harm exists and the very act of completing the one-time questionnaire indicates that the subject was willing to participate.

Federal *vs.* State Regulations

Federal regulations preserve a role for states in the regulation of research activities relative to informed consent. The federal regulations clearly state *informed consent requirements in this policy are not intended to preempt any applicable federal, state, or local laws which require additional information to be disclosed in order for informed consent to be legally effective* (45 CFR 46.116(e).

Additional Protections/Considerations

Informed consent is referenced in some state statutes addressing medical liability, mental health treatment, communicable diseases, acquired immune deficiency syndrome and human immunodeficiency virus infections, abortion, genetic testing, chemical dependency, etc. (Simon, Unutzer, Young, & Pincus, 2000). What these references have in common is the potential of sensitive information that could reasonably place the individual at risk of liability or damage to a person's financial standing, employability, and/or reputation. Review of research involving such topics is therefore required by an IRB. The IRB will determine the informed consent requirements for the specific project.

Institutional Requirements

Most universities and institutions that receive federal funding and conduct human research engage in a federal-wide assurance (FWA) with the Department of Health and Human Services. An FWA is an agreement to protect the rights and welfare of participants involved in human research as outlined in the code of federal regulations. Template consent forms that comply with federal, state, and institutional requirements are often available for researchers from their institutions. Often times, the wording is written in a simple question/answer format and conforms to local, state, and federal regulations.

5 | Clinical Trials: Design and Monitoring

Craig Tipton, BBA

Majid Moridani, PharmD, PhD, DABCC, FACB

A good clinical study is as good as its design and monitoring.

Introduction

In this chapter, we will discuss various types of clinical trials and important concepts in their design and monitoring. Retrospective, prospective, phase 0-4, dose-selection, and escalation trials will be discussed.

Food, Drug, and Cosmetic Act

In 1937, the United States experienced the "Sulfanilamide Disaster" in which about 100 people died after receiving tainted sulfa elixirs. The sulfa antibiotic, protonsil, had been discovered two years earlier, and though effective as an antibacterial agent, the deaths of so many attested to the need for strict controls on new drugs. In 1938, the United States Congress passed the Food, Drug, and Cosmetic Act. The Act was amended many times and lead to the creation of the Food and Drug Administration (FDA) as we know it today.

New drug formulations and medical devices must undergo rigorous testing in order to enter the U.S. marketplace. A new drug must demonstrate efficacy in humans and benefits that outweigh its adverse reactions. Some drugs, such as chemotherapeutic agents, can be toxic to humans, but because the end-result outweighs the risks posed to the patient, they can be used in the treatment of human diseases. In order to obtain the data to make these decisions, clinical trial medicine (CTM) has been developed to guide practitioners and researchers. Oversight and regulatory responsibilities fall upon the FDA.

Pre-Clinical Phase

In pre-clinical research, scientists attempt to develop new compounds in a laboratory. They rely on *in vitro*, *in-silico* (performed on a computer), and animal testing to investigate drug activity. Drug absorption, distribution, metabolism, elimination, and toxicity (also known as ADMET) is tested in various animal species. Drugs that demonstrate some efficacy in animal models and have a promising ADMET profile move to the next phase. Prior to any investigation in humans, the researchers file an Investigational New Drug (IND) Application with the FDA and form or locate an Institutional Review Board (IRB) to advise and direct the research on both an ethical and scientific basis.

Clinical Trial Medicine

Clinical Trial Medicine (CTM) should always ask definitive questions, such as, "In a group of 100 hypertensive patients in a double-blind randomized placebo-controlled study, will systolic blood pressure be reduced by 15% after administration of drug X for a minimum of six weeks?" CTM should never attempt to answer the question, "Does drug X cure hypertension?"

The root of CTM is the establishment of a causal relationship between the intervention and the outcome. To do this, researchers rely heavily on scientific rationale and ask questions, such as, "Are the results a reproducible indication of real efficacy or just background noise?" and "Is this a valid conclusion or are the data biased?" They conduct studies and observe the results. There is no room for data manipulation or variation from the trial design.

CTM is an inferential science. The researchers at best can only conclude that an outcome is likely or unlikely. They cannot claim that an outcome is certain, only that it is probable. It is impossible to test every human on the planet to find if a medicine is efficacious. Instead, we test representative samples of the human population and extrapolate the findings to the rest of population. There are many types of studies. Researchers test drugs, drug delivery systems, gene therapies, devices, surgical procedures, and psychotherapies. In addition to efficacy studies, they conduct studies to investigate dose, frequency of administration, and toxicity. While there are a variety of study types, they all follow strict clinical trial designs and answer critical questions about performance, such as:

- Are the results accurate?
- Has bias been avoided or minimized?
- Is the study question well formed?
- Are the patient's safety and rights protected?
- Is the intervention feasible for the patient?

The three main categories of clinical trials are descriptive studies, where researchers intend to identify a problem, associational studies, where researchers want to show a relationship between a factor and a condition, and explanatory studies, where a cause and effect relationship is established.

An example of each study type is illustrated in a research example that studies vitamin D deficiency in postpartum women. After recruiting patients with postpartum depression (as evidenced by an Edinburgh Postnatal Depression Score of nine or more), vitamin D blood levels are measured. This descriptive study described women with postpartum depression as having low serum vitamin D values. To demonstrate an association, the next step is to draw blood samples from postnatal women without postpartum depression as controls. If the control samples are high in vitamin D, we can claim that there is an association between vitamin D deficiency and postpartum depression. In the final study, causation is addressed when vitamin D is administered to women with postpartum depression to see if the depression resolves. If it does, a causal relationship can be claimed between vitamin D levels in postnatal women and postpartum depression.

Team Design and Monitoring

It works best if members of the clinical study team have predefined roles, so that the patient's safety is upheld and to ensure that the integrity of the data are maintained. Proper patient screening and selection can make or break a clinical study. Non-compliant subjects can skew the results. Unfortunately, data collection in a clinical study would never be perfect. Subjects drop out and the data from the early time points from the lost subjects loses its value.

Regulatory agencies, primarily the FDA, have oversight over drug development. The researchers are required to file an IND application and meet with the FDA for a pre-IND meeting and an end of phase II meeting. At these meetings, the FDA screens the study data looking for outliers and serious adverse events, as well as data that are "too perfect." Studies where no subjects missed a visit or data that is inconsistent with data from other sites in a multi-site study can be a red-flag for fraudulent findings. These findings can precipitate an audit and lead to the whole project being shut down.

Clinical trials frequently have a sponsor. The sponsor is the organization or company that is paying to develop the drug. The sponsor selects the qualified research personnel and sites, funds the study, files the appropriate regulatory paperwork, and is in charge of training critical personnel. The sponsor oversees and directs every aspect of the drug's development. Sometimes the sponsor will delegate the research operations to a research organization. This third party, the clinical research organization (a contract research organization), is expert in the intricacy of filing required paperwork and organizing a clinical research program. The medical monitor, who is generally a physician, oversees the medical aspects of the clinical research being performed. The research associate(s), as well as the investigator, site coordinators, and data managers, all report to the medical monitor and the sponsor. Each team member must conform to Good Clinical Practices (GCP). GCP carry the weight of law when a study is being reviewed by a regulatory agency or by a court of law. In short, they are the practices that researchers follow to ensure data integrity and ethical behavior.

Site Selection

Site selection is critical for the sponsor. The site for the study should not have too many other studies in progress. It should offer access to sufficient patients to conduct the work, and costs are always an issue. To ensure a diverse population, sponsors will often choose multiple sites in different geographic locations. Multiple site studies are more expensive to monitor than single site studies. In choosing a site, sponsors must consider how the site is going to recruit patients. Are they going to use a mass media campaign, or will they rely on physician referrals? These questions are answered up front by the sponsor and usually revolve around time and cost.

Once the team and IRB have been assembled and the study has been properly designed, clinical trials may begin, starting with Phase 0. The phases of clinical drug development are diagrammed in Figure 5.1 and explained in Table 5.1.

Clinical Trials Phases

Phase 0 is a relatively new concept in clinical trials, which was created in 2006 by the FDA to accelerate the development of new molecular entities. The objective of the trial is to investigate the pharmacokinetics of the drug in humans. The drug is administered at sub-therapeutic dosing levels, micro-doses not to exceed 100 µg or 1/100th of the effective dose as extrapolated from animal models. Ten to 15 healthy adult subjects are recruited to receive the micro-dose in a controlled setting. The study will gather basic data on how the drug is absorbed, distributed to the tissue, metabolized, and excreted. A general assumption is made that the relationship between the micro-dose and effective dose is linear from a pharmacokinetic standpoint. The following questions can often be answered by a phase 0 study:

- How long does the drug take to reach C_{max} (drug's peak concentration in the blood)?
- What is the drug's volume of distribution?
- Does it enter cerebral spinal fluid or only the interstitial space?

- Is it metabolized by the liver or does it spontaneously break down?
- Does it interact with P450 enzymes?
- What is the half-life of the drug?
- Is it eliminated by renal, biliary, or another route?

This phase can be critical in staging which drugs will be pursued.

Phase 1: In phase 1, 15-30 people will be enrolled. The average phase 1 trial costs approximately $500,000 and takes two years to complete. The primary purposes of this study stage are to assess the safety of the drug and to find the correct dosing range. These patient safety or pharmaco-vigilence studies look for adverse reactions to the medication. They can include side effects, such as nausea and/or QT interval prolongation. During this phase, the drug's benefits will be weighed against its costs to the patient. For instance, chemotherapeutic agents can be very difficult for a patient to tolerate, but the benefits outweigh the risk; therefore, even though the drug shows some side-effects, the trial will not stop. These types of scenarios must be thoroughly scrutinized by the IRB.

Dose escalation can be performed in many different ways. Initially, the drug doses should be investigated across age, race, gender, fasting/fed states, etc. The first dose begins at a fraction of the effective dose predicted in animals from the preclinical studies and is escalated until an effective outcome is reached in humans. The outcomes and the use of biomarkers should be defined prior to the start of the trials. Biomarkers come in three broad forms. The first type is the biomarker of disease, such as measuring TSH and free T4 levels in the patient's serum in the diagnosis of thyroid disease. A second type of biomarker is the kind that has pharmacological activity. An example of this type of biomarker would be looking at mean arterial pressure after the administration of a beta-blocker. The third type is a surrogate biomarker. This type of biomarker looks at ancillary attributes of a disease state or desired outcome because the actual outcome of interest cannot be quantified directly. For instance, researchers measure penile rigidity as a surrogate biomarker when attempting to quantify sexual arousal. Only about 70% of the drugs studied in phase 1 make it to the next stage of drug development.

Phase 2: In this phase, the researchers investigate their drug or device or diagnostic test in up to several hundred patients, and the research cost can be several million dollars. The patients studied in this phase have the disease or dysfunction under investigation. Phase 2 consists of two sub-phases: 2a and 2b.

Phase 2a provides the "proof of concept." This is the phase in which the sponsor finds out if the drug is actually effective in treating the disease in humans. Patients are randomized into groups. Some will receive the intervention, while others will receive a placebo or a sham device or procedure. In some situations, placebos and shams are replaced with the standard of care treatments because it would be unethical to put a patient on a placebo (e.g., replacing insulin with a placebo in patients with diabetes would be unethical). The patients will receive a treatment that is already considered as the standard of care, while the experimental group will receive the intervention alone or the standard of care plus the intervention. Phase 2a is solely concerned with the effect of the drug on the disease state and carries over the dosing data from phase 1 to answer the question, "Is the drug effective?"

Phase 2b, on the other hand, investigates the short term safety of the tested drug. The subjects enrolled in phase 2b have the disease. Up to several hundred patients may be enrolled in the study, and the effect of the drug will be measured against a placebo or a proven standard of care. The phase 2b study lasts six to 12 months because it is mainly concerned with short term adverse events. Only 33% of drugs tested at phase 2 will make it to phase 3.

Phase 3: Due to the huge cost increase in phase 3, not all drugs that successfully complete phase 2 will progress to phase 3. Phase 3 actively compares the investigative drug to existing standards of care. The clinical researchers consider available market share for the investigative drug to help make the decision to incur the costs of phase 3 investigations. This phase can enroll up to 1,000 patients and often lasts up to four years. The FDA requires a minimum of two trials before approving the drug. Phase 3 actively looks at safety, dose, and efficacy of the drugs. Phase 3 is a confirmation phase, as well as a testing phase. The purpose of the trial is to confirm that the drug is significantly efficacious compared to other standards of care and that the doses and timing are correct. Phase 3 is the last stage before the drug can be registered with the FDA and start generating revenue.

Endpoints in Design and Monitoring

Defining an endpoint is part of the testing procedure. The endpoints are divided to three groups: primary, co-primary, and secondary endpoints. A good primary endpoint should be responsive, sensitive, discriminating, and defined well before the beginning of phase 3. The investigator should ensure that sufficient data is collected to answer the question related to the primary endpoint. The generated data must be reliable, precise, and reproducible. The primary endpoint generally establishes a causal relationship between the intervention and the outcome. A co-primary endpoint may be necessary when the disease affects multiple measures, while a secondary endpoint may be ancillary data uncovered by the investigation that was not originally part of the study. For example, a secondary endpoint was reached with the drug minoxidil, which was originally developed to treat high blood pressure, but over the course of the investigation was shown to slow hair loss.

Upon completion of phase 3, the sponsor must file a New Drug Application (NDA) with the FDA. The FDA regulators will review the data from the previous phases and decide whether the investigational drug can be marketed in the United States. Approximately 25% of the treatments that enter phase 3 go on to phase 4.

Phase 4 can be initiated after drug approval by the FDA. At this point, the drugs are marketed. Phase 4 is referred to as post-marketing surveillance, and it never really ends. This phase includes many more patients than the previous phases. However, during this phase, the company that developed the drug is realizing a revenue stream. One of the most important aspects of phase 4 is that the patients are the ones reporting the outcomes. This is generally achieved via a website, a toll-free phone number, or mail services. The outcomes can be positive or negative. Some drugs that enter phase 4 will be recalled.

There are three classifications for recall. A "class I" recall is for products that will cause serious or fatal consequences. A "class II" recall is for drugs or devices that may cause serious, but reversible health effects, such as blindness that is not permanent and resolves once the treatment is stopped. A "class III" recall is for products that are not likely to cause immediate adverse health consequences. For example, propoxyphene with acetaminophen (Darvocet®) recently experienced a class III recall. The propoxyphene/NSAID combination was shown to cause a greater probability of addiction, but was not shown to be better than hydrocodone with acetaminophen. It ultimately rests with the manufacturer to recall a drug, since the FDA has no power to recall a drug or a treatment. The FDA does have the power, though, to enforce an injunction or restraining order, as well as seize or embargo a drug, as long as the courts have approved such actions via a civil proceeding. The FDA also has the ability to issue a "regulatory letter," which is more like a stern warning to the company.

Generics

Bringing a new drug or medical device to market is a long and costly process. And while it is critical for researchers to recoup their costs, their patent for these new medications only lasts for 20 years. The patent life begins when the company files the IND Application. Once this patent period ends, competitors are allowed to create drugs which are biologically equivalent to the original patented medication. These are termed generic drugs and are less expensive for the patient and usually preferred by insurance companies.

In 1984, the Food, Drug, and Cosmetics Act was amended to improve the time that it takes for generic medications to come to market. These drugs only have to prove bioequivalence to the original drug and do not have to go through all of the phases discussed earlier. Bioequivalence studies provide data that the generic drug, within a margin of error, behaves in the same way as the original medication from an ADMET and efficacy standpoint. The manufacturers do not need to file an IND or an NDA for generics. They instead need to file an Abbreviated New Drug Application (ANDA) with the FDA. Once the manufacturers of generics prove bioequivalence with the FDA and the patent on the original drug has expired, they are free to market the drug in the United States under the name of the active ingredient, such as simvastatin, but not Zocor®, the brand name for simvastatin.

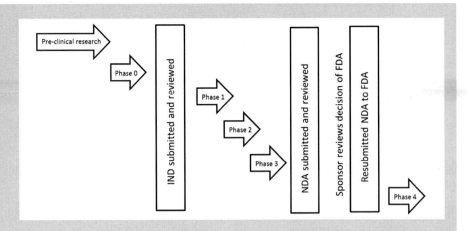

Figure 5.1: Various Steps in Clinical Trials Before Drug Reaches Market

Table 5.1: Summary Information on Various Types of Clinical Trial Phases and Their Success Rates

Phase	# of patients	Average Time	Average Cost	Focus	Probability of Success
Phase 0	10-15	6 months	$500,000	Pharmacokinetics	N/A
Phase 1	15-30	1 year	$500,000	Safety/Dosing	70%
Phase 2	<100	2 years	$1,000,000	Short Term Efficacy/Safety	33%
Phase 3	100-2000	3 years	$5,000,000	Safety, Dosage, Efficacy	25%
Phase 4 (post-marketing)	2000-200,000	4 years		Post Marketing Surveillance	N/A
Total (before the company can market drug)	Several Thousand	5 years	$7,000,000		3-6%

Minimizing Bias in Clinical Trial: Controls, Randomization, and Blinding

Bias

There are many different forms of bias, but ultimately a study is biased when outcomes do not reflect the true outcomes due to interference from some outside influence. For instance, if patients psychosomatically feel better because they think they are receiving the treatment, but they are really receiving the placebo, they are biased by the placebo effect.

In any clinical trial, there are three primary groups contributing to bias. The first group is the researchers, who include physicians, nurses, or anyone administering the intervention or designing the trial. The second group is the patients. Patients who know they were given a control behave differently than those who know they received the intervention. There is a subconscious tendency to conform to the expected outcome. The last group includes the data managers. They know which group is the control and which group is the experimental group, and there is always a fear that they may skew the data to make it conform to their preconceived ideas.

To minimize bias, three strategies are often employed: 1) to have controls as part of the study design, 2) randomization of the subjects to control and intervention groups, and 3) to blind the investigators, patients, and data managers to the group allocations.

Controls

Good control subjects are selected from the same population as the intervention group and only differ from the intervention group with regard to the drug they are receiving. The drug that subjects in the control group receive should look, smell, and taste just like the real drug. For a medical device or procedure study, the controls receive a sham. It looks like the real thing, but does not work.

Randomization

Bias is minimized when patients are randomly assigned to groups. Randomization creates study arms that are balanced against unforeseen risk factors. Randomization can be classified as simple or stratified. Simple randomization is just that, each person who meets the eligibility criteria is assigned a number and then placed in a group in a random fashion. Stratified randomization is used when there is some factor that could influence the outcome, for instance, age, body weight, or severity of a condition. Researchers use stratified randomization designs when they want to make sure all the oldest, thinnest, or sickest subjects don't by chance get assigned to the same group. Subjects are subdivided into homogeneous strata. Then the members of each stratum are randomly assigned to the various groups.

Blinding

To minimize various forms of bias, researchers use blinding techniques, so the people (investigators, patients, data managers) involved in the study will not have the opportunity to unduly influence a trial one way or the other. In the single-blind study, either the patient or the researcher is unaware of which intervention is the placebo or the active drug. A double-blind study is where both the researcher and the patient are unaware of the identity of the intervention. Most clinical trials are double-blind studies. There is also a triple-blind study that is gaining use in clinical trial design. This is where the patient, the researcher, and those who are analyzing the results are all unaware of which group is receiving the active intervention or placebo.

In order to use blinding techniques, researchers often split the trial into different steps. Then they will use different personnel along each step of the trial. When the researchers have fewer points of contact with the data gathering, patients, and the administration, there is less opportunity for bias to influence the outcomes. This technique certainly has its merits, but it also adds cost and time to the study.

Trial Designs

A study group or study arm is a group of patients that receives the same intervention(s) in the same sequence. Usually, it is done in a manner to minimize bias. Grouping can be done in many different ways. The patients can be assigned to the various groups by the researchers according to health states, age, gender, ethnicity, etc. This allocation can be balanced or unbalanced. Many times in larger studies, the intervention group or intervention arm of the study will be larger than the control group in order to test the intervention(s) against as many people and variations as possible. This would be an unbalanced grouping.

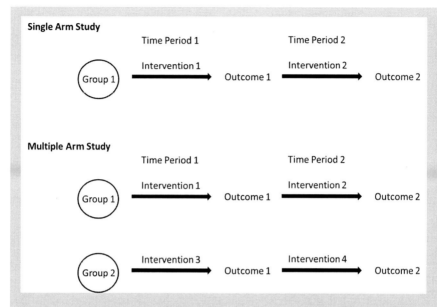

Figure 5.2: Schematic Representation of Single-Arm Study and Two-Arm Study

The study can have one or more than one intervention. The types and sequence of interventions may differ in the study. This figure shows two interventions.

There can be multiple groups or arms to a trial, as well (Figure 5.2). For instance, one arm could be an intervention that is the experimental drug at a 20 mg dose, while a second arm could be the intervention at a 50 mg dose, and the third arm could receive the placebo and create a control group. In "a within patient design," the trial is designed in such a way that the groups themselves are used to both accelerate the trial in terms of driving towards a definable endpoint, as well as minimizing bias. In short, patients receive more than one type of treatment. This can be achieved in many different ways. A cross-over study, for instance, switches which group receives the placebo and which group receives the intervention first. In this type of trial design, arm 1 of the study will start receiving the intervention and arm 2 will receive the placebo first (Figure 5.3). After a period of treatment and a wash-out period, arm 2 will cross-over to receive the intervention and arm 1 will receive the placebo.

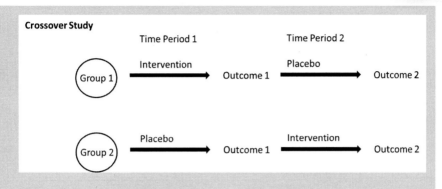

Figure 5.3. Clinical Trial Design in a Cross-Over Study

In a Latin Square design if there are n number of treatments, there will be an n number of parallel groups, creating n^2 number of trials. For instance, if there are two interventions with one placebo, that makes n, the number of arms, equal to 3 and three different time periods. So arm 1 will start with alpha treatment during time period one, move to beta treatment in time period two, and further move on to gamma treatment during period 3. Arm 2 will receive treatment beta during period one, move to treatment gamma during period two, and move to alpha treatment in the third period, and so forth for arm 3. Strictly speaking, this is the circular type of Latin Square design where beta always follows alpha, gamma always follows beta, and alpha always follows gamma. There is also a non-circular Latin Square where the type of treatment plan is randomized, and any plan can follow another. Depending on the study, either circular or non-circular may be appropriate. Some medications and treatments need to be administered in a sequential order, such as steroids should always be administered before antibiotics in cases of septic shock. However, the non-circular Latin Square is an excellent way to minimize bias in double-blind studies where the order of treatment is not critical.

While designing a trial, researchers often create caveats within the trial design to minimize patients' exposure to ineffective treatments.

This is a stop-gap measure that predefines a level of a disease state where patients must be removed from the study. An example of this would be diabetic patients receiving a new medication to manage their blood glucose levels. Prior to the intervention being studied in the patients, the researcher would define a range of blood glucose levels, a high level and a low level. If the patients cross either threshold, they will be removed from the study and placed back on their original therapy.

Dosing and Dosing Escalation

The purpose of dose escalation studies is to find an efficacious or therapeutic dose for humans and to characterize the range of possible effects that a new medication has to maximize the benefits of the therapy and minimize adverse reactions. An ideal medication is dosed infrequently, is easily administered (usually via the oral route), and is cost-effective to the patient. The main challenges that researchers encounter are risk-benefit ratio optimization and heterogeneity management (inter-individual variations).

The risk-benefit ratio optimization is very challenging when the goal is to find the dosing range in a myriad of patient types (e.g., patients of different ages, genders, with different levels of liver and kidney function) that gives the most therapeutic benefit with the least toxicity. This is accomplished by plotting dosing variation on a dose response curve as shown below (Figure 5.4).

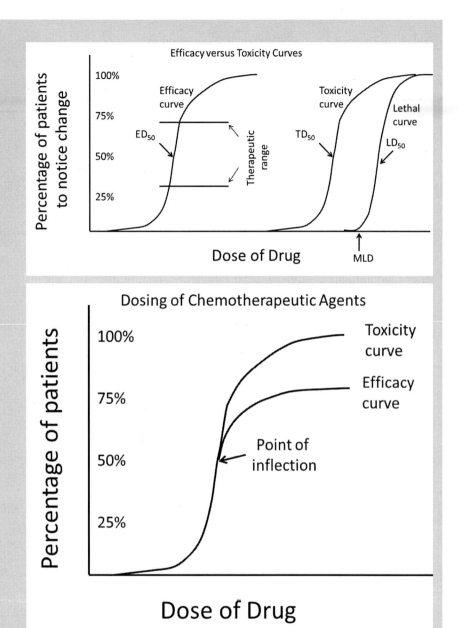

Figures 5.4a & b: Dose-Response and Dose-Toxicity Curves

The results of plotting dose vs. response give a sigmoidal curve, with dose as the independent variable and response as a dependent variable. As the dose increases, a larger number of patients will show a therapeutic outcome. Unfortunately, if the dose is increased too high, the toxicity increases, too. From the plot of these data points, researchers can find the median effective dose (ED50), which is simply the dose at which the desired effect occurs in 50% of the animals. This is not always the same as the median curative dose, though sometimes they are the same. Next, the minimum curative dose will be identified, which is the minimum dose to cure at least one animal, as well as the median toxic dose (TD50), which is the dose that causes toxic effects in 50% of the animals. Two very important points on this curve are the minimum lethal dose (MLD) and the median lethal dose (LD50). The MLD is the dose where at least one animal dies, and the LD50 is the dose where 50% of the animals die. For most new drugs, the researchers will graph both an efficacy and a toxicity curve. Ideally, there is a very wide gap between the two curves, this is the therapeutic range. For some chemotherapeutic drugs, the curves overlap. Here the researchers find the inflection point or dose where any additional dose quantity creates a marked increase in toxicity. The assumptions are that efficacy and toxicity are dose-dependent, that there is not significant variability in response by the patient, and that the dose response curve remains constant over time. This information is used to select a starting dose in clinical trial design of phase 0 or phase 1 studies.

The other important challenge is heterogeneity management. Heterogeneity is the variance observed between patients. This can include how quickly the patient metabolizes the drug, the patient's adipose tissue to muscle composition, age, genotype, or any number of other factors that affect the patient's response to an intervention. While this can be managed by grouping the patients, careful attention must be paid to all of the variables to ensure patient safety. Efficacy is always subordinate to patient safety.

In order to minimize patient risk and maximize safety, the data that are accumulated from animal research, as well as pharmacokinetic and ADMET information observed in Phase 0, will be used to identify a base dose to begin with in human trials. Then the dose escalation study will be performed in the patients in a timely and cost-effective manner. This is achieved in a few different ways. The first is the single ascending dose (SAD) method. This type of dose escalation uses a dose per group per time period, and then escalates the dose in the next group for the next time period, and so forth. Each group is monitored closely for efficacy and ADMET. Although this method is the safest approach in determining the dose range, it is also the most costly and time-consuming method. The next method is the multiple ascending dose (MAD), in which a variable of escalated doses are evaluated in the first group for the first time period, say 10 mg, 20 mg, and 30 mg, the next group in the next time period will then begin with a 40 mg, 50 mg, and 60 mg dose. This escalation is continued until the drug's dosing profile is mapped, but ended prior to significant toxicities being observed, as predefined by the IRB. Across both of these types of escalation, researchers will be testing the doses in the fasting and fed states of the patients in order to observe how the drug is absorbed under different conditions and in combination with different food types, such as protein and fat-rich foods.

Types of Studies

There are many different ways to create a better understanding of patient health, in addition to the randomized double-blind study. Each of these study types has its own strengths and weaknesses (see also Chapter 2).

A *retrospective study* looks backward through time at medical records for a distinct group of patients and divides the groups to compare the subsets and their respective outcomes. For instance, employees at a textile factory could appear to have a high incidence of skin cancer. If the researchers split the employees into groups of those who work with heavy dyes and those who only work in the office area in the same factory, they can then look at the incidence rates of cancer within the subsets of employees to determine if there is an association between the dyes and cancer. Retrospective studies are generally inexpensive, can take less time than other types of studies to conduct, and are excellent for determining relative risk. However, the researchers may find that the data are incomplete. In addition, the determination of a causal relationship is impossible to prove in a retrospective studies.

A *prospective study* is fundamentally the same as the above, except that it looks forward in time. While this type of study certainly takes longer and is more expensive than a retrospective study, researchers will have the ability to gather the data they choose to study.

A *case series* is an observational study where researchers select subjects based on their known medical problems and track them based on treatments and/or outcomes. This type of study can be retrospective or prospective and has been used as a cornerstone of medicine for hundreds of years. For example, a new diabetic medication comes to market and a physician prescribes it for a few of his patients with diabetes. He monitors their responses over the next few months or years to observe whether their conditions improve. The physician would be studying a case series. There are many problems with this type of study. One problem is selection bias, where the physician subconsciously chooses the healthiest patients to include in his case series, and then assumes it is the new medication which is helping the patient, when in fact the new medication has only marginal benefits.

Other types of **observational studies** are cross-sectional, case-control, and longitudinal studies. *Cross-sectional studies* observe a population or subset of a population at a distinct point in time. This study is concerned with describing an entire population. By contrast, a *case-control study* is only concerned with distinct groups, such as IV drug users or liver transplant patients, and then compares their health outcomes to a control group's outcomes. The former two observational studies can be considered snapshots of populations, groups, and their outcomes. Conversely, a longitudinal study observes groups or populations across long periods of time. *Longitudinal studies* may observe the same people for many decades, gathering data about health decisions and how those decisions correlate to outcomes.

Cohort studies are a subset of longitudinal studies where small populations, a cohort, are tracked over time. The essence of a cohort study is the analysis of risk factors that the small group experience and how these factors translate to outcomes over time. The correlation of risk factors to outcomes can be used to calculate absolute risk of contraction within a population.

Randomized controlled trials (RCT) are the focus of this chapter. This type of trial randomizes the subjects into an intervention group and a control group, and then quantitatively measures the patients' outcomes. RCT are especially important to healthcare because they are the most likely to show a causal relationship between an intervention and an improved health state. The RCT can further be subdivided into *before-after studies and cross-over trials*. The difference between the two subsets of RCT's is how the arms of the study are treated with regard to the intervention being studied. If the intervention and control arms start and end the trial with no change in therapy or placebo, it is a before-after study. If the arms switch between receiving the intervention and placebo sometime during the trial, it is a cross-over study. The crossover study is particularly effective in proving a causal relationship, as well as minimizing bias, and is therefore used extensively in clinical trial design.

Incidence and Prevalence

While many may use the words incidence and prevalence interchangeably, they are different. Disease incidence is the measurement of disease occurrence over a period of time, whereas disease prevalence is a measurement of disease for a population at a point in time. Measuring incidence is asking the question, "How many people will contract pneumonia this year in our community?" Measuring prevalence is asking the question, "How many people have pneumonia in the community?" If a pharmacist wants to stock sufficient vaccine for his community, he should look for incidence. If he wishes to have a treatment plan for the community, he should look at prevalence. In thinking of these measurements, the clinician should also be concerned with reliability, validity, accuracy, and precision to determine the strength of the measurements.

Reliability, Validity, Accuracy, and Precision

Reliability: If peanut butter is rubbed into a patient's hair and the patient's hair grows where formerly it would not, a researcher might postulate that peanut butter makes hair grow. If peanut butter makes hair grow in every bald person, the treatment would be reliable. Reliability is the repeatability of the experiment and can be quantified with Cronbach's Alpha. Cronbach's Alpha is usually calculated with a computer due to its complexity and is a measure of correlation between questions or trials within an experiment. The closer the value is to one, the greater the correlation of consistency between trials.

Validity, on the other hand, is a measure of the strength of the conclusions and hypothesis. In short, is the conclusion true or false? Within validity, there are further measures to find how valid an experiment is in relation to the outcomes. Internal validity measures the strength between the experiment and the observed outcome. So did the peanut butter cause the hair growth or was it just coincidental? If internal validity is high, then there is a greater probability that the independent variable is responsible for the dependent variable. External validity is concerned with being able to translate this experiment to the greater population. If the researchers can rub peanut butter on anyone's head and generate greater hair growth, then there is external validity. Construct validity covers how the experiment is designed. If the question is about peanut butter and hair growth, and the researcher measures self-confidence as an outcome instead of actual hair length, then there is no construct validity. Conclusion validity is the measure of the relationship between the outcome and the statistical methods used to come to the conclusion. Are there confounding variables that were not accounted for in the final measurements? Were the correct statistical tests used?

Accuracy and Precision: Accuracy is the ability of a measurement to be correct, while precision is the degree to which something can be measured. For example, accuracy would be measuring a hair to be six inches long when the hair is actually six inches long, not five inches long. Precision on the other hand is being able to distinguish between a hair that is six inches long and one that is 6.1 inches long.

Summary

For better clinical trial design and monitoring, specific attention should be given to the type of questions that a clinical trial intends to answer. Planning should be devoted to building a research team and selecting the most appropriate study design to answer the posed question. The study team should work diligently with the IRB, draft a consent form, carefully select inclusion and exclusion criteria, choose the sites for the study, comply with regulatory requirements, avoid bias by including a control group, randomization, and blinding techniques in the study design, and keep accurate records of the study.

6 | Clinical Research and Ethics

Osvaldo Regueria, MD

Walter Bridges, MD

Mubariz Naqvi, MD

Introduction

Ethics is the systematic study of values that guide us to see the difference between right and wrong. It is not the same as morality that usually relates to how a person is brought up and influenced by religion and culture. Ethics is also different from laws and regulations that proscribe conduct. Can an Alzheimer patient give consent to enroll into a clinical trial? Can a researcher perform testing in addition to what is described on the consent form on collected samples without getting additional consent from the study subjects?

Human subjects should be used in clinical research only when there is no other means (e.g., tissue culture or animal studies) to answer the clinical question. In the 1970s when AIDS research was being conducted on animals, there were inquires from patients who wanted to volunteer for the studies. They were desperate and did not want to wait for animal studies, which would take several years to complete before human trials could be started. However, data for the development of a vaccine were not available. Human trials without at least some animal data would have been unethical. The risks would have far outweighed any potential benefits.

Recently, an AIDS vaccine trial being conducted in Africa was questioned about why the study was not being carried out extensively in other countries. In the early 1980s, animal rights activists successfully lobbied for a ban on the sales of animals from shelters to medical schools in some cities in California. When asked about alternatives, the animal-rights activists suggested human "volunteers" from the prison population be used (Rutecki, 2007).

These are just a few examples of the ethical dilemmas that face clinical researchers. This chapter attempts to answer some of these questions and review the basic ethical principles involved in human clinical research.

Historical Perspective

One of the earliest mentions of ethical principles is in the Hippocratic Oath, which requires the physician to "do no harm." This principle is at the heart of clinical research ethics. Subject safety is paramount. Although it cannot be eliminated, risks to the participants must be minimized.

Due to atrocities committed by Nazi physicians in World War II and other abuses mentioned elsewhere in this book (Willowbrook hepatitis study and Tuskegee syphilis study), several codes of ethical conduct have been developed to protect participants in clinical research. The Nuremberg Code, Declaration of Helsinki, the Belmont Report, and others are the foundation of clinical research ethics. These documents delineated the basic ethical principles of **autonomy, nonmalficence, beneficence,** and **justice.**

Autonomy relates to informed consent and requires full disclosure of the study purpose, methods, benefits, and risks. **Nonmalficence and beneficence** require that a study maximize benefits and minimize risks to the subjects. **Justice or fairness** relates to equitable selection of participants.

Tenets of Clinical Research

Out of these basic principles, seven main tenets of clinical research were developed. These include: 1) social and clinical value, 2) scientific validity, 3) fair subject selection, 4) independent review, 5) risk-benefit ratio, 6) informed consent, and 7) respect for potential and enrolled subjects (Perlman, 2004).

Social and clinical value implies that a study should have a significant value or benefit to society or the participants in regard to their disease. **Scientific validity** relates to how a study is designed. There should be a clear scientific objective with acceptable methods. **Fair subject selection** defines who should be included. Enrollment should not be based on economic or vulnerability factors. Subjects should benefit from the study and risks should be minimized. Even with a favorable **risk-benefit ratio,** the risks of a new or investigational drug cannot be completely eliminated. Risks can be physical, mental, economic, or social. Benefits should be maximized and outweigh risks.

Independent review requires an institutional review board (IRB) and data safety monitoring boards. These committees are involved in design of the study and continued monitoring. **Informed consent** demands full disclosure of benefits, risks, and alternative therapies, and must be voluntary. More extensive discussions about the IRB and informed consent are in Chapters 3 and 4. **Respect** for potential and enrolled subjects includes the right of privacy, the right to a change of mind, the right to be told about new information that arises during the study, and the impact on participant welfare.

Data safety and monitoring boards (DSMBs) work in conjunction with IRB's to monitor ongoing participant safety (Silverman, 2007). Board members include statisticians who advise clinical investigators. The board periodically reviews study data, adverse events (AEs), efficacy, and progress. Data are evaluated for quality, completeness and study site performance, protocol adherence, and compliance. DSMBs are not required in all studies. Retrospective chart reviews and phase 1 and 2 studies don't require DSMB monitoring, although phase 1 and 2 trials do require a safety monitoring plan. Studies using collected tissue samples also do not require DSMB monitoring.

In the past, most clinical trials were done mainly in academic institutions. Currently, many clinical trials are sponsored by for-profit companies. Researchers and clinicians are routinely paid for enrollment of participants, while IRBs are often paid to review the data. This has the potential to alter objectivity and introduce bias.

The number of clinical trials has increased dramatically in recent years. This stresses oversight processes and has increased pressure on researchers to recruit potential study participants. With this increase in publications, there has been a significant increase in retractions of publications due to misconduct. An alarming number of article retractions have been due to duplication, data fraud, the inability to independently reproduce results, plagiarism, and failure to receive IRB approval (Budd, Coble, & Anderson, 2011).

Practical Encounters with Ethical Issues in Clinical Trials

Some research studies pose no more than a "minimal risk" to the patient. Many other clinical research studies are straight-forward and require the subject to receive one mode of treatment or another. While enrolling patients for a research study, the investigator will undoubtedly come across situations common to all patients. These situations are anticipated and discussed in the consent form. Inevitably in a pluralistic society such as ours, unique situations will arise that cannot be foreseen in the planning of a consent form.

Informed Consent

The concept of a "true" informed consent requires an understanding by the subject (or legal guardian, if a minor) of the elements of the research, risks involved, possible outcomes, benefits, and alternative treatments (Pedroni & Pimple, 2001). If the subject is a competent youngster (seven years old or older, but may vary by state), an assent should be obtained after providing similar, if simplified, information (see also Chapter 4). The patient (or legal guardians), the hospital, and the outpatient clinic must receive a copy of the signed consent forms.

> **Example:** We ask that a copy of the consent form be present in the patient's chart prior to carrying out any

chemotherapy orders. Many of the recent protocols require re-consenting at different stages in the study, and if missed, a patient may receive treatment for which they have not truly given their consent. In some circumstances, this may legally constitute assault and battery of the patient. Should the patient suffer severe side effects from an unauthorized treatment, the investigator may be subject to penalties and medical-legal exposure. Sanctions from the state medical board and loss of licensure can result.

Recent immigrants to the U.S. may have little or no understanding of English. Many come from lower socioeconomic groups and have little education. While the most common second language in the U.S. is Spanish, over the past few years, a significant number of patients come to our clinic from Africa, Asia, and other remote geographical locations. A true informed consent is difficult to obtain with a language barrier, but remains essential. It is the investigator's obligation to ensure adequate translation services are provided.

The availability of various telephone translation services with bilingual native speakers is invaluable. We must be able to rely on the translation being an accurate interpretation of our statements, even though we are unable to discern so at the time of consent. Therefore, at our institution, we have designed a "simplified consent form" that includes all the required elements of consent translated to the patient's native language by a certified translation service. Each of the consent elements is referenced to the section of the English consent provided at the time of consent. This allows the patient or parents to read them later, after they have a better command of the English language. This process also assures us that the phone translator uses these precise central themes in their discussion with the subject.

Special Situations, Parental Rights

In addition to language, social or religious concerns may be of enormous importance to the subject and should not be ignored by the researcher. If there is a strong likelihood of side-effects to the treatment and the subject would find them objectionable because of his/her beliefs, this must be clearly discussed and documented prior to administration of any therapy.

In clinical practice, if the local institution is not able to satisfy the needs of the patient (for example, Jehovah's Witnesses who refuse transfusion of blood products), patients should be referred to an institution that can provide these services (a clinic that practices 'bloodless medicine' with plasma extenders, etc.). At a minimum, the availability of such centers must be made clear to the patient so as to have true consent.

In situations more relevant to daily clinical practice rather than a research study, even though the majority of treatment consents state the parents have the right to request treatment and to stop treatment at any time, in practice this is not always the case. If in the opinion of the physician, the child, as a result of withholding treatment, is at high risk of serious sequelae or death if the treatment or procedure is not carried out, the state can automatically take over as temporary custodian of the child. The physician is then obligated to treat the child regardless of the parents' feelings and over their objections. This is a highly undesirable and utmost unpleasant situation for all parties involved. It places an enormous stress on the parent/caregiver relationship and can result in significant loss of trust, anger, and resentment.

A case in point is that of Jehovah's Witnesses and their prohibition of blood product administration. In the case of chemotherapy treatments, most patients require either red blood cell or platelet infusions during the first few weeks of treatment. The need for blood products is much lower in the later stages of treatment, and almost nil during the maintenance phases. Prior to enrolling in a study, it is imperative that the possible need for blood product transfusion be discussed at length in realistic terms. Adults may refuse potentially life-sustaining treatments for themselves at any time, even if it would result in their death. However, minors are seen in a different light by law (in Texas), and parents do not have the right to refuse transfusion of blood components in an overt life-threatening situation. Physicians are required by law to transfuse the child, even if they have to obtain an emergency court order to do so.

There are now centers that specialize in the practice of "bloodless" medicine. The use of plasma expanders and others agents is maximized, and only when absolutely necessary is a transfusion given.

The extremely low levels of hemoglobin at which these centers allow their patients to drop are well beyond what the ordinary physician is accustomed to and would probably be objectionable to a majority of them. In our experience in the case of Jehovah's Witnesses, their local representatives are a great help in locating these specialized centers.

Similarly, in the case of a child with a malignancy, if parents request the administration of chemotherapy to be curtailed, the physician may be obligated by current laws to continue treatment. The anger, frustration, and loss of trust of the parents towards the caregiver can be avoided if the parents understand this aspect of the consent form/law before treatment is initiated. Since most of the treatment's alternatives involve similar if not identical drugs and risks, parents are usually quite understanding and accepting of this aspect of treatment.

Consents within Consents

In research studies that involve patient tissues, several studies may be conducted simultaneously or in the future with specimens. Tissues may be sent to different testing centers as part of different research studies. These "satellite" studies must be clearly listed in the body of the consent form. At minimum, they must be referred to by study number or title. The patient must be made aware of the different studies embedded within the main study, and each should be referred to by study number and/or title in the consent form.

Patients must agree, commonly in the form of yes/no questions, to the use of their tissues for research dealing with their disease (for example, leukemia), other types of similar diseases (for example, leukemia subtype), or totally different diseases (for example, diabetes or heart disease). Furthermore, how long specimens/tissues can be stored and the type of testing the patient allows to be carried out must be clearly delineated. The risk of disclosure of a patient's identity through processing of these specimens and the right to withdraw consent of specimen testing/banking and the procedure involved (i.e., the person to contact to withdraw) must be clearly stated.

Reaching Legal Age While Under Treatment

Situations arise where the patient enrolled as a minor with parental permission becomes an adult, while still taking part in a research study. The investigator must respect the wishes of the newly emancipated patient as those of any consenting adult. If they request to not continue in the research study, this must be respected. This includes the use of any specimens, banked tissues, or genetic material previously submitted while they were underage.

In Texas, another somewhat unique situation arises when a pregnant female who is a minor is emancipated during her pregnancy (emancipated minor), and consents to take part in a research study. Her consent may no longer be valid after delivery because she reverts to minor status at that time. This applies to non-study therapy, as well. Each state interprets this particular situation differently, so it is necessary for investigators to be familiar with the laws in their state. Valuable information is usually available from the risk-management office at your institution.

Disclosure of Errors

Medical mistakes are more common than we would all like to admit. To the patients in a research study, mistakes in dosing of therapeutic agents or other errors in treatment may carry significant immediate and future consequences. It is imperative the subject be informed at the earliest opportunity of the nature of the mistake and possible consequences. Failure to do so is unethical, but will also likely lead to anger and resentment on the part of the patient towards the caretaker upon discovery at a later date. Irreparable damage to the patient/caregiver relationship and trust is likely. A timely, honest, and sincere discussion of the events with the family will help overcome this eventuality. The investigator will often be surprised by how very understanding and forgiving of errors patients and their families are as long as they are treated in an honest fashion with full disclosure.

Inadequate Specimens and Additional Procedures

Specimens obtained for the sole purpose of research, with no immediate clinical value to the patient, should be obtained as an extra aliquot at the same time the procedure is regularly scheduled for clinical purposes. The procurement of the additional tissue/sample for these purposes must be included in the consent. Under no circumstances should an additional procedure be conducted for the sole purpose of a research study. For example, if a bone marrow aspirate is collected, but it is only sufficient for clinical diagnosis and treatment, it would be unethical to re-aspirate the marrow for the sole purpose of obtaining a specimen for a research study. The additional specimen should have been obtained at the time of the original bone marrow aspiration. If the additional specimen is a study requirement, the study should be terminated and the patient/subject informed of the reason.

Some studies are designed to obtain a specimen for testing levels of a drug. These are commonly paid subjects and the previous discussion would not apply to them.

Source of Supplies/Medications and Reliability of Products

Many oncology investigations are conducted by one of the major study groups, such as the Children's Oncology Group (COG) or Southwest Oncology Group (SWOG), where the study materials are pre-approved by the study group and local IRB for quality and performance. Independent studies must ensure the same quality of materials and assure an adequate supply be available throughout the expected duration of the study.

In the event a medication that requires the administration of an "antidote" is being studied, a supply of the latter must be secured prior to the administration of the treatment. An example of this would be a patient receiving high dose methotrexate, with leucovorin being administered as an antidote at a prescribed time.

Should an unforeseen shortage of a medication occur, the patient must be informed of any changes in scheduled treatments. Any substitutions may fall outside of the consent signed at initiation of treatment. A signed addendum to the original consent may be necessary if the treatment agent was not included in the original consent. The local IRB should be notified of these arrangements and approve of the revised consent form prior to the treatment substitution. In such cases, emergency or expedited IRB approval is available under most circumstances.

What if A Better Treatment Becomes Available?

If during an investigation new information becomes available that shows superior results to those expected in the ongoing study, the patient must be informed immediately. Termination of the current study and transfer to the superior, proven treatment would be the ethical option. If a significant difference in outcome between arms of a protocol is suggested by the available clinical and statistical data, it is mandatory that the patients be transferred to the arm with the advantageous outcome.

If a treatment or procedure is poorly tolerated by a patient, the caregiver may need to re-evaluate the patient individually and determine if stopping treatment would be the best and most ethical alternative for the patient.

Protection of Subject's Privacy

The safe-guarding of protected personal information is not only of utmost importance, but is required under the mandates of HIPAA (see also Chapter 3). An investigator must be familiar with these requirements. Violations will result in significant fines to the investigator. The persons or entities that may have access to this information (e.g., COG, SWOG, NIH) need to be clearly delineated in the consent form.

Patient Harm Resulting From Study Involvement

While some side-effects will decline when treatment agents are decreased or discontinued, some significant side-effects may persist and become permanent. Treatment for these side-effects or compensation for the afflicted patients is not commonly paid for in clinical trials. Patients must be aware of these facts.

In the event a patient is or believes he or she has been harmed by being involved in a research study, a person or entity to contact for assistance should be clearly stated on the copy of the consent form given to the research subject. Many institutions have patient representatives that may assist in evaluating subjects' concerns and help arrange a meeting with the parties involved.

Integrity of Data

Unethical manipulation of research data or the outright invention of results has damaged the reputation of many researchers in recent years. Unfortunately, a few unscrupulous individuals have been able to rise to high professional positions based on falsified data prior to being exposed as frauds. Even more significant is the possible exposure and harm that may come to the individual patients treated according to fallacious data. A case in point was the implication of vaccines as the cause of subsequent development of autism. The allegation has now been shown to have been unfounded and the original claims retracted (Greenhalgh, 2010). The parental concerns motivated by this fraud have resulted in the refusal of thousands of children to receive vaccines that would have protected them against childhood illnesses. Some of these diseases were once almost eradicated, but recent outbreaks have been reported (Iannelli, 2009).

Vignettes and Analysis

Informed consent: A 72-year-old Alzheimer patient has given consent to be enrolled into a clinical study involving an investigational drug for memory. The patient is unable to give information about the purpose of the study or methods involved.

This case involves informed consent and most probably requires a surrogate decision-maker to give consent. The surrogate's decision must be based on the risk-benefit ratio and what is in the best interest for the individual. This would also apply to individuals with other causes of diminished decision-making capacity, as well as children. In children, if they are able to understand the purpose, risks, and benefits of the study, their opinion and assent should be considered.

Right to Withdraw: During a clinical trial involving stem cell transplantation, a significant number of patient withdrawals occur. This could harm the study statistically if more withdrawals occur. The principal investigator wants to modify the informed consent form to make discontinuing or withdrawing from the study a **mutual** decision requiring both the participant and the researcher to agree.

This would violate the principle of autonomy. Consent must be voluntary, and the study participant must be able to withdraw from the study without impediments, reprisals, or compromising future care.

Risks vs. Benefits: A research study involving a new antibiotic for meningitis is being compared to the standard antibiotic treatment for meningitis. The standard antibiotic dose in the study however, is less than the accepted optimal dose in the standard treatment. This study was stopped due to the potential risks to the participants who had a life threatening illness and were receiving suboptimal doses of antibiotics.

The risks outweighed the potential benefits.

Unexpected Adverse Events (AEs): During the conduct of a clinical trial involving an investigational drug, the adverse events in the investigational group were significantly higher than the control group. Should the study be stopped? Should the study participants be informed of the adverse effects?

Depending on the severity of the AEs and potential risk to the investigational group, discontinuation of the study should be considered. Participants should be informed of the events and allowed to choose whether to stay in the trial or not. Ethically, when statistically significant data, whether positive or negative, are noted, discontinuation of the clinical trial should be considered and the patients transferred to the best-outcome alternative.

Full Disclosure: A smoking cessation study involved ten sites, with five sites serving as the 'control' (no intervention) group. The study was presented to participants as a smoking cessation program with different interventions conducted at the five 'intervention' sites. Participants were not informed that this was part of a research study.

When questioned, researchers contended that to inform participants of the research aspect of the project would potentially alter their responses to follow-up surveys, thus altering the results. Another aspect discussed was whether having only intervention groups (no controls) would help justify non-disclosure.

Non-disclosure is never justifiable, and the subject has the right to full disclosure prior to agreeing to participate in a research study.

Conflict of Interest: An editor of a research journal receives an article that is in the same area of research as the editor's colleague. The editor alerts his colleague about the pending publication and also delays the review of the article.

This would illustrate a case of favoritism and certainly a conflict of interest.

Right to Determine Use of Subject's Tissues: After completing a study which involved collection of tissue samples, a researcher wants to do additional testing not explicitly described in the initial consent form. Does the investigator need to get a new consent form from each study participant for the additional testing?

Most IRBs will require an additional informed consent or, at minimum, a signed addendum to comply with the right to full disclosure.

7 | A Basic Protocol

James K. Luce, MD
Candace A. Myers, PhD

A study protocol is a recipe for performing an experiment. It clearly states the research question and describes every step taken to conduct the study. A competent reader should be able to understand how to carry out all the details of the study and locate the needed materials in order to reproduce the study results. The protocol should support the feasibility of answering the research question and is necessary to obtain the IRB approval to conduct a study in humans.

Some institutions have a specific format for a protocol. Check with your IRB administrator. A number of resources were considered in developing this discussion. A basic protocol typically consists of the following elements:

1. Descriptive study title
2. Investigators and their contact information
3. Introductory summary
4. Background and justification

5. Objectives and hypothesis
6. Materials and methods
7. Risks
8. Power analysis and plan for statistical analysis
9. Data management and safeguards for subjects
10. References

Descriptive Study Title: Compose a concise, accurate, and descriptive title for the study.

Investigators and their Contact Information: Identify the principal investigator. List his/her name, degree(s), position, departmental and institutional affiliation, address, email address, and a reliable phone number. List similar information for each co-investigator and study team member. You may also briefly describe the contribution each person will make to the study.

Introductory Summary: Include a brief summary or abstract that describes the study.

Background and Justification: This element will cover an interesting and compelling description of the clinical condition being studied, current treatments, the limits of current knowledge, previous research, the significance of the subject area, a justification for asking the research question, and a description of the contribution the results will add to current knowledge. You may summarize animal studies, laboratory data, pharmacology, toxicology, and potential adverse events. Technical information about the test article is needed. Explain what variables you plan to study and why they are important. Develop the study's question(s). Key references should be cited. A thorough literature search will supply the information needed. Try to limit this section to two or three pages.

Objectives and Hypotheses: In this section, the investigator defines the objectives and the hypotheses for the study. List each major objective and the specific aims that will allow you to reach each objective. Objectives must be specific, measurable, attainable, reliable, and time-limited. The specific aims are the two or three study activities that are planned to fulfill the objective.

Reword the objectives as hypotheses that will allow statistical testing. For instance, if the objective is to identify biomarkers of endothelial damage in the urine of adolescents with Type 1 diabetes mellitus (T1DM), the specific aims might be to: 1) collect urine from eligible subjects, 2) quantify present level of endothelial damage, 3) analyze urine for potential biomarkers, and 4) correlate potential biomarkers with endothelial damage. The research hypothesis is: Urinary biomarkers are positively correlated with endothelial damage in adolescent T1DM subjects. The null hypothesis is: Urinary biomarkers do not correlate with endothelial damage in adolescent T1DM subjects.

Material and Methods: In the material and methods section of a protocol, you explain what will be done, by whom, how, where, when, and using what? The methods are the procedures necessary to achieve the objectives of the study. The source of all services (e.g., lab analyses), materials, and equipment should be listed, so that someone trying to replicate the study can locate the same items, repeat your work, and get approximately the same results. These are the tactics of the research. The following criteria should be discussed in this section:

- Setting: Clinic, outpatient, hospital.
- Study Design: What you will do – retrospective chart review, prospective study, cohort, cross-sectional, case-control, cross-over. Justify the design.
- Sampling Design: Describe the randomization procedures, control group vs. intervention (test) group(s).
- Sample Size: Demonstrate sufficient power, and discuss the feasibility of conducting the study in your setting.
- Study Population: Justify the population choice (age, gender, and ethnicity). Research conducted with subjects in a protected group, such as children, prisoners, pregnant women, people with impaired decision-making ability, and those who might be in a position to be coerced due to their social status (such as an employee) require special

justification. List inclusion and exclusion criteria. State the amount of the stipend or incentive to be offered to study subjects, and how it will be paid. Explain how payments will be prorated if subjects withdraw before they complete the study.

- Recruitment and Consent: Describe recruitment strategies. Describe where potential subjects will be approached, and who will obtain consent. Describe what will be explained to subjects during the consent process, and how you will ensure that subjects understand the protocol. Describe risks and benefits, including possible loss of privacy, confidentiality, and record anonymity.

- Benefits and Harm: Describe potential benefits and possible harm to subjects. Benefits may be direct, physical, psychosocial, or they may be collateral benefits to society. Potential harm could be physical, psychosocial, or loss of an opportunity for an alternative intervention that might be advantageous to the subject. Provisions for medical or other professional interventions in the event of adverse events must be described.

- Study Groups: Describe the control and experimental groups. Interventions can be therapeutic (using drugs, devices, procedures) or diagnostic, and include blood draws, imaging, and biopsies.

- Test and Placebo Substances: Describe the test and placebo substances, any analytical tests, proper storage, plans for distribution of test and placebo substances, and how you will account for the substances.

- Study Duration: List the anticipated study duration in your setting.

- Data Collection: Describe data collection sheets, variables to be collected, coding for samples, and sample handling procedures. List chemical analyses, interview questions, and observation techniques. Itemize the study activities.

- Procedures for Laboratory Analyses, Measurements (Units), Apparatus/Equipment Used: Supply references for the published methods. Provide the source (company, city, state, and country) of all reagents and equipment used in the study.

- Study Timetable: List the anticipated study start date and completion date. Provide a graphic timetable with notations of major study activities. Clarify that you have sufficient resources to complete the study in the specified time period.

Risks: If the research will involve more risk than the subject would normally encounter in ordinary daily life or during a routine physical exam or psychological test, the protocol should itemize the 'greater than ordinary' risks. Procedures to minimize risk as much as possible should be described. Potential risks can be physical, psychological, social, economic, legal, and loss of confidentiality. Discuss how the potential benefits of the research or importance of the knowledge make the risks reasonable.

Statistical Analysis: List the descriptive statistics you plan to summarize, and the statistical tests you plan to conduct. It is always a good idea to get your biostatistician's input during the drafting of the protocol. She/he may also need to conduct a power analysis to justify the sample size.

Data Management: Describe the storage of data collection sheets, entry of data into a computer system, and de-identification of individual subject records, if appropriate. Where will records be stored and how will they be protected? What steps will be taken to maximize privacy and confidentiality of medical information? How long will records be kept before they are destroyed? Will identifiers be attached to data, or will data be coded or unlinked?

References: The bibliography will include key articles to support the claims you made in the Introduction and Background and the methods you plan to use. It may cite some landmark papers, but most of the articles should have been publications within the last five to ten years. Always cite the original reference that presents the data to support the claim.

Appendices: You may need to include specific methods for analyses, copies of surveys/questionnaires, flyers or advertisements used for recruitment, and copies of data collection forms.

8 | Data Collection

Paul Tullar, MD

Robert P. Kauffman, MD

Careful collection of individual data points and their safe retention is the most basic of research functions. The conduct of the study with skillful attention to every detail of the protocol will ensure that all the steps that came before and all the steps that come after are worth doing. The fruits of the labor of careful data collection are basic and irreplaceable.

What data to collect are defined by the protocol. Who collects the data is limited to the trained study team described in the IRB-approved records. Raw data collection is usually best done on paper. Thought should be given to the format and flow of the data collection sheet to ensure ease of collection and to prevent missed entries. A data collection sheet with a blank for every variable to be collected is a convenient way to make sure all pieces of data are collected for each consented subject.

Keep study documents organized in one place, and keep them safe from loss. They are primary source documents and prove that the data were collected. Study records should be kept under lock and key in a centralized Clinical Research Unit, or in the principal investigator's office. Records must be available for audit at any time. Storage should be independent of the individuals conducting the projects such that when individuals leave the employment of the sponsoring institution, relevant research materials can easily be accessed by succeeding study team personnel. Check with your institution or agency about their retention policy. Some identifying information (master sheets) can be destroyed as soon as they are no longer needed in an effort to preserve the privacy of study subjects. At our institution, records are kept for three years after the study was reported (manuscript printed).

Efforts should be made to limit the number of records that contain protected health information (PHI). Investigators often maintain a master list that links the subjects' names or medical record numbers to unique study subject numbers. A good practice is to store the master sheet separately from the other study documents, and to identify all the other records by subject number only. No data containing PHI should be visible to anyone other than the approved study team in order to protect confidentiality of the research subjects.

Data include demographic information, time of day, date, laboratory test results, observations, films, scores, and any measurements taken as part of the data collection process. For example, if the chemistry lab records the temperature of their lab or refrigerator or the lot numbers of the reagents they use, these are data to be maintained (if they are germane to the experimental design).

Data are typically transferred from the paper data collection sheets to an electronic file maintained in a secure password-controlled computer or computer network. An electronic database or spreadsheet (MS Excel) is best prepared by or with the close cooperation of a statistician. The design should take into account the eventual analysis of the data. A general convention is that the individual subjects are listed on the vertical or "Y" axis, while the dependant variables (test results for each subject) are listed along the horizontal, or "X" axis.

Table 8.1 is an example of an MS Excel spreadsheet.

Table 8.1. Example of an MS Excel spreadsheet.

Subject	Age	BMI	Parity	Gest_ Age	Category	Gallstones	Glucose	Insulin	Leptin
P03	28	37.3	2	36	Obese	yes	85	21.1	45.7
P04	20	22.9	0	32	Lean	no	88	10.6	54.0
P05	24	20.1	2	34	Lean	no	76	2.0	6.0
P06	27	29.4	2	36	Over-weight	no	78	12.5	37.4
P08	21	21.9	1	11	Lean	yes	80	7.0	26.6
P09	38	33.0	2	32	Obese	no	83	9.9	47.2
P10	21	48.1	1	12	Obese	no	79	5.7	17.6

When working with electronic files, it is a good idea to back-up your files on a regular basis.

Most variables can be categorized as 'continuous' (numbers), 'nominal' (qualitative, yes or no, red, yellow, or black), or 'ordinal' (1st, 2nd, 3rd, etc.). The timing of an event can be another important variable. Think about how much precision is needed in the record. Is 1 PM, 2 PM sufficient, or does it need to be 13:52? Alternatively, some may need to record time of a second event in relation to an initial event, such as 0 minutes, 60 minutes, etc.

Be consistent in defining your 'dictionary' or 'code book' of responses for your nominal variables. (For example: 1 = 'yes', 2 = 'no'). Keep the dictionary somewhere attached to the spreadsheet, so the person entering the data and any reader looking at the raw data can easily decode the values. Define missing values and 'outlier' data points you want to exclude. Missing data and excluded data have implications for the statistical conclusions of the study. Follow a scheme and be clear about what data are entered and how they are entered.

Enter one datum result per cell in the electronic spreadsheet. For continuous data, enter the same number of significant figures for each subject's record of a particular variable. Make sure you conform to significant figure conventions when data are manipulated.

Most research studies encounter missing data points. Sometimes the subject does not want to answer a question on a survey. They may consider the question too sensitive. Missing data points can sometimes have serious implications for the statistical analysis and interpretation of the study. Incomplete data may be problematic in several ways. If subjects vary considerably in responses, even a few missing data points may cause mis-estimation of effect. Other problematic difficulties introduced by missing data points include reduction of sample size that may lead to loss of statistical power. Multivariate analysis (analysis of several variables at the same time on the same subjects) requires complete data on all subjects included in the analysis.

At times, a researcher may wish to exclude a data point as an outlier. The assumption is that some misstep during data collection occurred and resulted in an unreliable value that does not add valid information to the study. Any excluded outliers need to be accounted for, both on the data collection sheets and in the spreadsheet. The circumstances leading to the exclusion need to be clearly recorded.

There are a number of ways to deal with missing data. If the data are continuous, with a normal (Gaussian) distribution, a straightforward way to deal with one missing value is to calculate the average and insert it for the missing result. You might just remove the subject from consideration for that variable, and re-calculate the average without the missing subject. You will need to modify the number of included subjects as an "N" for each variable, and state that there was no obvious systematic reason for a few missing data points.

Following data collection and entry into the electronic spreadsheet, the statistician will receive the spreadsheet and the protocol. The analyses described in the protocol should be performed using a statistical package, such as SPSS (Statistical Packages for Social Sciences), STATA, or MedCalc. In addition to summarizing the results, the statistician will provide the printed output to retain with the study records.

Study team authors are now ready to scrutinize their results and see what conclusions they can draw.

9 | Introductory Statistics for Clinicians

Majid Moridani, PharmD, PhD, DABCC, FACB

Rajiv Balyan, DVM, MSc

Medical science is an ever-changing field. **Statistics** are critical for understanding the disease prevalence data, epidemiological reports, and to derive a correct interpretation from data collected in clinical trials. It allows us to reach meaningful conclusions that we can apply. For example, if body temperature rises in disease X and drug B reduces it back to normal in one person, we cannot conclude that drug B is really helpful in decreasing temperature if the drug is only tested in a single patient. This is because the assessment of the drug effect in a single patient cannot always be generalized. However, if the body temperature of 100 patients is lowered by drug administration and appropriate statistical analyses are performed, then we can confidently conclude that drug B will produce a **clinically relevant** decrease in body temperature when it is administered to a patient with an elevated body temperature. By utilizing descriptive and inferential statistics, we can predict if drug B can reduce temperature in another group of patients suffering from fever. The statistics can further help in determining the appropriate dose and interval of drug administration.

Descriptive Statistics

Descriptive statistics help in understanding the basic features of the data, and summarize the data collected in a study. For example, a graph can be used to represent deaths due to type II diabetes in Texas in the last 20 years. The descriptive data might be presented in graphical or tabular form, so the overall outcome buried in raw data can easily be grasped.

The **frequency distribution** of data can be presented as a histogram, bar-graph, pie-chart, dot-diagram, or simply in tabular form. The **bar-graph** (Figure 9.1) is used when data are qualitative, such as categorical data (e.g., color formation in gram staining of bacteria: i.e., pink or violet) or quantitative (numerical) with discrete intervals (something which can be counted in whole numbers, like the number of beds in a hospital, deaths due to tuberculosis in a given year, etc.). **Pie-charts** can be used for the same types of data.

A **histogram** (Figure 9.2) is used to depict a continuous quantitative variable, like hemoglobin levels in blood. Observations are continuous because they can assume any value in a range, such as 8.1, 8.2, 8.3 or 8.4%. Each column represents an interval of variable, such as 6.0-6.9, 7.0-7.9, 8.0-8.9, and 9.0-9.9. The height of the column indicates the frequency distribution in that specific interval. A **line-graph** is created by joining all the observations with a straight line or fitted into a curved line. If there are a small number of observations, a **dot-plot** is a good choice, and each dot indicates an observation. The **scatter diagram** represents two different quantitative variables associated in an observation. The position of an observation on the graph indicates the magnitude of each variable.

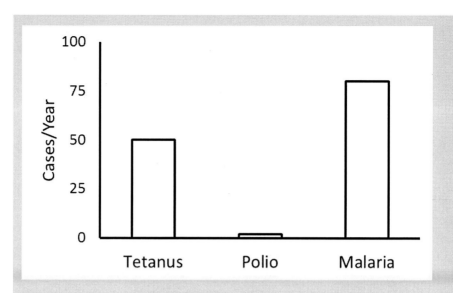

Figure 9.1: Bar-Graph Summarizing Number of Deaths Due to Infectious Diseases in a Given Year

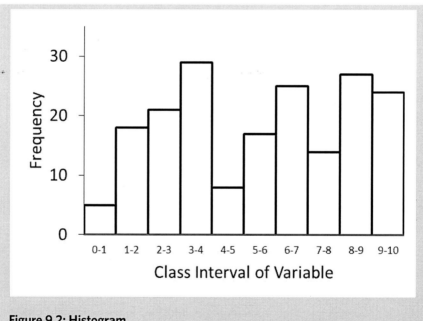

Figure 9.2: Histogram

Types of Variables

Variables are quantitative or qualitative. Quantitative variables can be continuous or discontinuous. **Continuous** variables involve all theoretically possible values between an upper and a lower point (limited by the precision of the analytical method and the instrumentation, i.e., 7.2 feet or 100 mg/dl are continuous values). **Discontinuous** or discrete variables are identified by a specific integer (whole number). For example, the address of a house in a block or a woman's number of live births are discrete variables. They must be an integer, like five, six, or 105, and can never be a fraction. Qualitative or **categorical** variables are nominal or ordinal. A **nominal** variable can be divided into distinct categories, but there is no inherent order. For example, skin color could be white, black, brown, or yellow. There is no way to rank nominal variables. **Ordinal** variables do have an order between categories, though the interval or distance between each order is not uniform, for example, the four stages of melanoma.

Mean, Mode, Median, Range, Variance, and Standard Deviation

The descriptive statistics also employ certain numerical measures, which tell about the central character of a data set in a quantitative manner, and the 'normal' value of the data. These values provide an idea about where most of the values are positioned in a given data set. They are also known as **measures of central tendency** and **measures of dispersion**. The measures of central tendency include: mean, median, and mode. The measures of dispersion include: range, inter-quartile range, variance, standard deviation, coefficient of variation, and standard error of means.

Measures of Central Tendency

The **arithmetic mean** (usually designated as the **mean**) is the most popular measure of central tendency. It is the sum of all observations divided by the number of observations in a data set. To calculate arithmetic mean of 2, 10, 12, 14, 16, 20, 24, 28, 32 and 38, the sum of the numbers is divided by the number of values 196/10 = 19.6.

The **geometric mean** is used when there is a huge variation between observations in a category. For example, if we have numbers like 1, 10, 10,000, and 30,000, an arithmetic mean will not provide an accurate representation of the observations in a data set. Here, one needs to calculate geometric mean for central tendency, which can be calculated from the log value of the observations, the arithmetic mean of log values, and finally by calculating the antilog of the arithmetic mean. For instance, the geometric mean in the above example can be calculated as following: (log 1 + log 10 + log 10,000 + log 30,000) /4= (0 + 1 + 4 + 4.48)/4= 2.37. The antilog of 2.37 is 234, which is the geometric mean of the data set for the above four numbers, which is more realistic than the arithmetic mean of the same numbers.

Median is the middle number in a group of observations arranged in ascending order. If we arrange 11 boys in increasing order of their heights, then the height of the boy in the sixth position will be the 'median.' In this case, there will be five boys taller than the middle boy and five boys shorter. Median indicates that an equal number of observations are distributed on either side of the median value. If there is an even number of observations, the median is the half-way point between the two central values.

Mode is the observation value that has the most frequency of occurrence in the data. If observations within a group include two, three, four, four, four, and five, then the mode is four. A data set containing a single mode is called **unimodal**, while a data set containing two modes is called **bimodal.** For instance, the biomodal distribution of pharmacokinetic half-lives in isoniazid therapy indicates the existence of slow acetylators and fast acetylators in the general population. In normally distributed data, mean, median, and mode are the same. If data are skewed, such as when the distribution curve is not bell-shaped, and the peak is inclined towards one side and tailing at the other side, the mode will be the peak (where most of the values are located), the mean will be shifted towards the outliers, and the median will be between the mode and the mean (Petrie & Watson, 1999).

Measures of Dispersion

Measures of dispersion provide information about the spread of values in a data set across the central value. It is the indication of variation in observations, which include range, inter-quartile range, variance, and standard deviation. The **range** is the difference between the smallest and the largest values. The major critic of range is that it depends solely upon the extreme values in the data set, which does not provide any information about the rest of the data. For instance, if we study the HDL cholesterol levels in a group of 100 healthy adults and calculate the range from these values, the range will tell only about the difference in cholesterol levels in two individuals and nothing about cholesterol levels in the rest of the group. Hence, range is not considered as a very useful measure of dispersion.

Inter-quartile range provides information about the spread of the central 50% of the values. It is calculated by subtracting the individual value in the 25th percentile from the individual value in the 75th percentile. Inter-quartile range is a better indication of dispersion because it provides information about the distribution of half of the values across the middle of the data set. Inter-quartile range is not affected by extreme values. Percentile is calculated by considering all the observations as 100%. A percentile is the value of an observation greater than certain observations, for instance, at the 20th percentile, 20% of the data points are located to the left in ascending order. The 25th percentile is also called the **first quartile (Q1)**; the 50th percentile is the **second quartile (Q2)**; and the 75th percentile is the **third quartile (Q3)**. The second quartile is the same as the median.

Variance is the measure of deviation of individual values from mean value. To get a better understanding of how values are spread in a data set, calculate the value's distance from the mean by subtracting calculated mean from each observation. Variance provides information about how far each observation is located from the arithmetic mean in either direction. An average of these deviation values provides a clear idea about the spread of the values in a data set. However, the problem is that the sum of all deviations from the mean in a data set is always zero. This is because the sum of the positive deviations from the central value equals the sum of the negative deviations. To overcome this problem, all deviation values are squared. The square of both positive and negative values is always positive. The average of squared deviations indicates the variation in the data across the mean, and is termed the **variance**. However, there is still a problem in using variance as a measure of dispersion. This is because the squared values are bigger than the individual values (or smaller if the values are less than 1); hence, it is difficult to comprehend and apply. To overcome this problem, the square root of variance known as the **standard deviation (SD)** is generally used to provide a sense for the measure of deviation of the individual values from the mean value (Daniel, 2009). SD is close to the observations in magnitude and free of a positive or negative sign. The SD provides a numerical range within which most of observations fall in a normally distributed data set (Figure 9.3). The SD is represented by the Greek letter σ (sigma). One σ range from the mean (μ) covers 68% of the central observations. Two and three σ from μ covers 95.4% and 99.7% of the observations. To have the central 95% and 99% values, the σ is multiplied by 1.96 and 2.58, respectively. Table 9.1 summarizes the range of values derived from mean and SD.

Table 9.1: Summary of Range of Values Derived From Mean and SD

Limit	Distribution of values
$\mu \pm 1\,\sigma$	68 % of values across mean
$\mu \pm 1.96\,\sigma$	95 % of values across mean
$\mu \pm 2.58\,\sigma$	99 % of values across mean

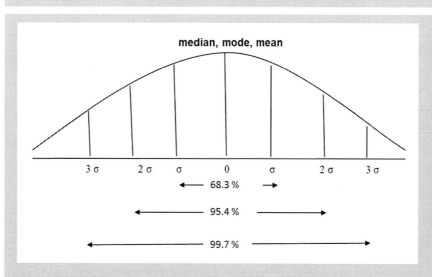

Figure 9.3: Bell-shaped Curve or Normal Distribution Plot

SD is the most commonly used measure of dispersion in presenting clinical findings, assuming the data distribution follows a Gaussian normal distribution. Bar-graph depictions of two different groups with the mean and SD (error bar) allow a quick decision about the existence of a significant difference between the two groups. If the error bars representing the SD values of the two groups overlap, the groups are not significantly different (Figure 9.4).

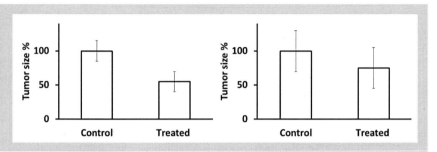

Figure 9.4: Left - SD Error Bars Do Not Overlap - Groups Significantly Different. Right – SD Error Bars Overlap - Groups Not Significantly Different (Sample Size N=3).

Both the SD and mean carries the same units. To nullify this change, occasionally some researchers use another dimensionless measure known as **coefficient of variation (CV)**. It is the SD expressed as the percentage of mean. Due to a few theoretical complications, CV is not used widely.

Another important measure of dispersion is the **standard error of the means (SEM)**. The SEM provides information about the dispersion of sample means of different groups across the population mean and how deviated the sample means are from the population mean. The SEM is calculated as $\sigma/\sqrt{n}$ for a population, where n is the number of observations and σ is the population SD. SEM is also known as simply **standard error** or SE.

Both SD and SEM are used in medical journals to show the variation in data points around a mean. SEM is always smaller than the SD and can give a false sense of low variation within samples, making groups look significantly different when they really are not. The P value provides a true measure of significance (Norman & Streiner, 2009).

Remember that SD is a measure of the scatter of the data around the mean. It is an average measure of deviation of each individual data point from the mean of that data. It can be used to construct reference intervals that indicate the range for most of the data in a population. However, SEM is a measure of the precision of the sample means as an estimate of a population mean. It can be also used to define the confidence interval for the sample means.

Probability

How can we apply the descriptive information to a larger group? Suppose, one has access to the health-related data of 300 children in the three to five years age group in Sudan, and 8.4% of those children are affected with hypopituitarism. How can one apply this information to estimate the prevalence in two million children of that age group in Sudan? It is not feasible to gather information about two million children due to time, cost, and logistics limitations. That is where one needs **inferential statistics,** which helps in applying the finding of a smaller sample size to a much larger population. The downside of such an estimation is that one cannot be completely confident about the prediction we make about the larger population based on the findings from a smaller sample size. Therefore, there is an element of doubt associated with the inferential conclusion. One can be confident only to a certain degree. This degree of confidence is termed **probability**. The probability is one of the most widely used applications in statistics. Probability means what are the chances of a favorite event occurring in a set of events. For instance, if we count 100 cars on the road, how many of those are Hondas. For calculating probability, first the possible number of outcome is determined, followed by determining the chances of a favorable outcome to occur in a study. Probability is also defined as the number of favorable events occurring in a number of experiments performed under similar conditions. The value of probability ranges from 0 to 1. The 1 value means unity, an absolute certainty of occurrence of a favorable event. The 0 value means null, an absolute certainty of non-occurrence of a favorable event.

There are two fundamental rules in calculating probability: the addition rule and the multiplication rule. The **addition rule** states that if two events are **mutually exclusive,** meaning that if one event occurs, then the other event cannot occur (for instance, a coin flip cannot produce a 'heads' and a 'tails' for the same flip), then the probability of either event to occur is the sum of the two individual probabilities. The **multiplication rule** states that if the two events are **independent,** meaning that the occurrence of one event does not affect the other event in any manner, then the probability of both events to occur is the product of the individual probabilities. For example, a person suffering from bradycardia may or may not be afflicted with lymphosarcoma. There is no relation between the two conditions, hence they are independent. There is one other kind of event known as **conditionally probable**. If there are two events A and B and the occurrence of B depends on A, then the probability that both A and B will occur is the probability of A times the probability of B, provided that A has already taken place. For example, a person infected with HIV later dies from AIDS. Here, the two events of HIV infection and death due to AIDS are conditionally dependent. The person's death from AIDS may occur only after HIV infection, but not in the absence of HIV infection. Thus, these two events are **conditionally probable** (Armitage & Berry, 1994).

The probability of a continuous random variable could be graphed to determine the probability of specific intervals. When all these points are joined, the line forms a bell-shaped curve and the graph is called a **probability distribution graph**. If the bell-shaped curve is symmetrical with the peak of the graph at the center indicating highest probability at the mean, then this distribution of probability is called a **normal distribution**. This graph could be used to compare two groups consisting of a random variable or to answer specific questions, such as whether a particular event will happen or not in a given condition. For example, we want to know if drug A is better than drug B in treating arthritis. To answer the question, we first draw a hypothesis.

A **hypothesis** is a statement we wish to prove in a study. It should be well defined in terms of scope and depth of the study, and should be clear from any obscurity or vagueness. There are two types of hypotheses, a **null hypothesis** and an **alternative hypothesis**.

Null hypothesis (H_0) states the negative or default condition. For example, "There is no difference in the prevalence of breast cancer among Chinese and American women." The **alternative hypothesis** (H$_1$), also known as the research hypothesis, is the opposite of the null hypothesis and states that there is a difference between the two groups. In the previous example, the alternative hypothesis is, "There is a difference in the prevalence of breast cancer between Chinese and American women." Here, the investigators do not know if American women are more prone or less prone to breast cancer compared with Chinese women. They just believe that there is a difference. Since there are only two groups, the appropriate statistical test needed to answer this question is a **two-tailed test**. If the investigators know the trend of the difference (for instance, the prevalence of breast cancer is either more or less in American women compared to Chinese women), then they would need to use a **one-tailed test**. When using one-tailed tests, information based on scientific evidence that the trend exists in a certain direction is required. When uncertain, a two-tailed test should be used to answer the question. For more information on one-tailed and two-tailed tests, see useful online websites at the end of this chapter.

After formulating a hypothesis, a **standardized score** or a **z value** is calculated using the mean and the variance. It is the expression of an observation in terms of a SD. The z value of +1 means the observation is one SD more than the mean. Based on z value, the probability could be obtained from a table. The z value determines if we can accept or reject the null hypothesis at a specific **significance level** or with a certain probability (P), such as 0.05. The P value of 0.05 is a universally accepted standard in biological sciences. If we accept the null hypothesis at a 0.05 significance level, it means we are 95% confident that the null hypothesis is true, and there is no significant difference between the two groups. However, there is a 5% uncertainty about this conclusion. This is the price we pay for using the conclusion formed from a sample of observations to make a prediction about a population. Similarly, if we fail to reject the null hypothesis at the 0.05 significance level (that means we accept the alternative hypothesis at $P = 0.05$), then we are 95% confident that there is a significant difference between the two groups. The 0.01 and 0.05 are standard cutoffs for comparing data in medical sciences. It is usually written as $P < 0.05$, indicating that we are more than

95% confident about the conclusion or that more than 95% of the observations will fall under our stipulation.

Student's T-Test

Student's t-test can be used to accept or reject a hypothesis. The test was proposed by William Sealy Gosset, who used the penname 'student' for publishing his work because his employer did not want him to publish, thinking that his statistical method should remain a trade secret. The Student's t-test can be a **one-sample t-test**, if you are using it to ascertain a fact about the test group, or a **two-sample t-test**, if you wish to compare the means of two groups. For a two-sample t–test, it is assumed that the variances of both groups are equal. If the variances are different, a modified version of the t-test, known as **Welch's t-test,** is applied. Variance is assumed to be equal for one-tailed and two-tailed t-tests, and the software commonly used today performs all the calculations. If variances are not equal, there is a correction option in the software.

If the same subjects are used as both the control and test groups, a **paired t-test** is used to compare the data. For instance, in a drug trial of a novel treatment for diffuse cutaneous leishmaniasis, lesions in the same patients before and after drug administration are measured, and a paired t-test is used to assess the drug efficacy. If there are reasons to believe that the underlying assumption of t-test, i.e. normality and randomness, are not met, then the **Wilcoxon rank sum test** (for paired groups) or **Mann-Whitney** U **test** (for unpaired groups) should be substituted for the Student's t-test.

Type of Errors, Sample Size, and Power of Analysis

It is possible to make an error when accepting or rejecting the null hypothesis. Data analysis may suggest that the null hypothesis is not true and that there is a significant difference between the means of two groups. As a result, the null hypothesis would be rejected. However, what happens if in reality there is no significant difference between the two groups. Hence, we commit an error by rejecting the null hypothesis when it should be accepted. This is called a **type I error**. On another occasion, the data analysis may suggest that the null hypothesis is true (no significant difference between the means of the two groups), but in reality there is a significant difference between the two groups. In this case, a **type II error** is committed by accepting the null hypothesis when it should have been rejected. The probability of committing a type I error is denoted by α, and the probability of committing a type II error is known as β. Both α and β should be determined at the beginning of an experiment. The β is usually kept small and expressed as $1 - \beta$ (usually expressed in terms of percentage). The value for $1 - \beta$ is used in determining sample size and the **power** of the test. The higher the power of the test, the greater the chance of getting a correct conclusion from the study (Petrie & Watson,1999). It cannot be increased to 100% because there will always be some uncertainty associated with statistical methods. For clinical trials, the power analysis is usually estimated at 80%.

The sample size calculations and power of the test calculations for a clinical trial design are affected by the expected effect-size, the hypothetically or realistically expected standard variation in the study group, type I error (α), and type II error (β). As a general rule, the larger the effect size and the smaller the variation in the effect size, the smaller the sample size. When type I and type II errors are small, the sample size must be larger (Table 9.2).

Table 9.2: Types of Errors

	Statistics conclude	In reality	Error
Null Hypothesis (There is no difference)	rejected	should be accepted	Type I error (α)
	accepted	should be rejected	Type II error (β)

Statistical Significance and Clinical Significance: What Is the Difference?

Before blindly following the recommendations of statistical tests, we need to understand the difference between **statistical significance** and **clinical importance** or **biological significance**. If a sufficiently large sample size is studied, small differences between treatments may prove statistically significant. Suppose we compare the efficacy of drug X and drug Y in lowering blood pressure. Drug X costs $1/day and drug Y costs \$5/day. Drug X leads to an average 10 mmHg drop in blood pressure, while drug Y reduces it by 12 mmHg. This difference may be statistically significant if a large sample size is chosen, but the difference may not be very important clinically, and may not be worth spending the extra money on drug Y. Clinical significance, which is defined by outcome and endpoints, is more important than statistical significance (Armitage & Berry, 1994).

Analysis of Variance (ANOVA)

Student's t-test is useful for comparing the means of two groups. What if there are more than two groups? If we conduct t-tests for every possible combination of two groups, we will increase the type I error (α), and it is likely to get statistical significance merely by coincidence. For instance, if we wish to compare four groups, there are 16 possible ways to compare the groups using t-tests. If the significance level is set at 0.05, one out of 20 comparisons will arrive at a conclusion that there is a difference between two groups by chance alone. The **analysis of variance (ANOVA)** is a method of comparing the means of more than two groups, which can overcome the limitations discussed above.

When comparing two groups, we can also use the F-test. The null hypothesis is that the variances of the two populations are equal. If the ratio of variances is equal to one or less, depending on the degree of freedom (which relates to the sample size), then the F-statistic, indicated on the F-distribution table, would indicate that the null hypothesis should be accepted (no significant difference between the two groups). The ANOVA uses the same principles as the F-test to compare the means of more than two groups. In an ANOVA, the null hypothesis is that all the observations come from a single population (the variation between the group means would be the same as the variation between observations within the groups), and the group means are not different. The alternative hypothesis is that there is more variation between group means than within the groups. If the variance ratio is equal or greater than a tabulated value at a given degree of freedom, the null hypothesis is rejected, which means that at least one group mean is statistically different from another group. If ANOVA indicates there are no significant differences between groups, no further statistical investigation is needed. If ANOVA reveals that there is a significant difference between groups, a post-hoc analysis is required. Post-hoc tests include **Scheffe's, Tukey's, Bonferroni's,** and **Duncan's** tests. For non-parametric comparisons, tests such as **Kruskal-Wallis one-way ANOVA** and **Friedman two-way ANOVA** can be used (Portney & Watkins, 2009).

Chi-Square Test

The t-test and ANOVA are used to compare arithmetic means or quantitative variables. When dealing with qualitative and categorical variables, the chi-square test is appropriate. Instead of comparing the means, the test compares the proportions of cases expressing a certain quality among levels of a given factor or among combinations of levels of two or more factors. The variables are binary (i.e., there are only two mutually exclusive possibilities for a variable). As with the t-test, a null hypothesis is established that there is no difference in the proportion of two groups, or there is no association between the two variables. From a 2 x 2 contingency table of proportions, expected frequencies are calculated. A t-value is calculated using observed and expected frequency values. The corresponding P value is obtained from the table. The decision to accept or reject the null hypothesis is based on the P value. In addition, the chi-square test of goodness of fit is used to test the hypothesis that the total sample N is distributed evenly among all levels of the relevant factors. If the expected frequency of the data is less than five in any of the cells in a Chi-square table, **Fisher's exact test** should be substituted for the Chi-square test. Table 9.3 gives an example of Chi-square analysis.

Table 9.3. Example Chi-square Analysis to Evaluate the Effectiveness of Drug B Compared to Drug A

	Positive Response	No Response	Total
Drug A	20 (a)	40 (b)	60 (a+b)
Drug B	14 (c)	6 (d)	20 (c+d)
Total	34 (a+c)	46 (b+d)	80 (a+b+c+d)=N

$X^2=(ad - bc)2/[(a+b)(c+d)(a+c)(b+d)] \times (a+b+c+d) = [(20\times6)-(14\times40)]2/[60\times20\times34\times46] \times 80$

X^2= 8.25, the result simply indicates that drug B is more effective than drug A.

Measurement of Association

When studying the pattern of occurrence of a disease in a specific population, some investigators may focus on subgroups of the population, such as who was exposed more to the disease, identifying new cases at a given time, and the total number of cases in the population. These types of information can be used to establish a relationship or association between the population and the disease. The measures of this association could be used to predict the chances of occurrence of a disease in a population in a given geographical area and to determine what proportion of that population is affected by the disease. These measures include **relative risk, incidence rate, odds ratio, hazard ratio,** and **correlation coefficient.**

Certain factors may influence the outcome of a variable and may increase the chances of occurrence of the disease. Such influencing variables are known as **risk factors**. For example, smoking is a risk factor for lung and oral cancers. The group of subjects exposed to the risk factor is more susceptible to develop cancers compared to a non-exposed group. The **ratio of probability** for the manifestation of a disease in an exposed versus a non-exposed population is termed **relative risk (RR)**. In a household where parents smoke, kids face a relative risk of harm from second-hand smoke compared to kids whose parents do not smoke. The RR risk may assume any value between zero and infinity. The RR of one indicates that exposed and unexposed populations have equal chances of acquiring the disease, and that the 'risk factor' is not really a risk factor. An RR value greater than one indicates that the exposed population is more likely to develop the disease.

The RR value is an indication in a prospective study of something that is going to happen in the future. The entire population is divided into groups depending on their exposure to risk factors. However, in retrospective studies and case-control studies, the investigators deal with individual subjects who have either exhibited or not exhibited the disease. The ratio of cases having the disease to cases not having the disease is called the **odds ratio (OR)**. The word 'odds' carries the same meaning as the usages in "what are the odds of rain today" or "what are the odds of winning the lottery." It is an indication of the risk factor on subjects in a retrospective study. Like RR, the OR can assume any value between zero and infinity. An OR value of one indicates that the risk factor was not associated with the disease, and both exposed and non-exposed individuals manifested the disease in the same proportion. An OR value of greater than one indicates more chances of the disease in individuals associated with the risk factor compared to individuals not associated with the risk factor. Similarly, an OR value of less than one indicates less chances of the disease in individuals associated with the risk factor.

Clinical studies of diseases generally deal with prevalence, epidemiology, and how effective a particular treatment is in preventing or treating a disease (Aitchison, Kay, & Lauder, 2005). For instance, consider a clinical trial studying the effect of a drug in reducing the death rate due to renal failure. One group receives the treatment and the results are compared to a placebo or untreated group. Assuming that the probability (relative risk, rate) of death after completion of the study is 0.05 and 0.30 for treated and untreated groups, respectively, then $0.30 - 0.05 = 0.25$ provides the estimate of reduction in death rate due to the drug treatment. This is known as an **absolute risk reduction**. Another commonly used measure of reduction is the **relative risk reduction**. The decrease in disease occurrence is determined relative to the probability of disease occurrence in a control group. Using the previous example, the relative risk reduction will be $(0.30 - 0.05)/0.3 = 0.83$ or 83% reduction, while the absolute risk reduction was 25%. Thus, the relative reduction rate is a more sensitive measure of treatment efficacy. Table 9.4 compares odds ratio, rate, absolute risk reduction and relative risk reduction.

Table 9.4: Odds Ratios, Rate (Relative Risk), Absolute Risk Reduction, and Relative Risk Reduction

	Condition		
	Absent	Present	Total
Control Group	5	40	45
Treatment Group	25	35	60
Total	30	75	105

	Rate	Risk Ratio	Odds	Odds ratio
Control Group	0.89	1.52	8.0	5.71
Treatment Group	0.58		1.4	

Rate = proportion in the group with condition present.

Rate [Control Group] = 40/45 = 0.89 means 89% are affected in control group.

Rate [Treatment Group] = 35/60 = 0.58 means 58% are still affected in treatment group.

Risk ratio = Rate [Control Group]/Rate [Treatment Group] = 0.89/0.58 = 1.52 means that the control group is 52% more affected than the treatment group.

Odds [Control Group] = Present [Control Group]/Absent [Control Group] = 40/5 = 8 means that from every 9 = (8+1) people in the control group, 8 are affected.

Odds [Treatment Group] = Present [Treatment Group]/Absent [Treatment Group] = 35/25 = 1.4 means that from every 2.4 = (1.4 + 1) people, only 1.4 are affected after treatment.

Odds ratio = Odds [Control Group]/Odds [Treatment Group] = 8.0/1.4 = 5.71.

Absolute risk reduction = Rate [Control Group] – Rate [Treatment Group] = 0.89-0.58 = 0.31 or 31%.

Relative risk reduction = Absolute risk reduction/Rate [Control Group] = 0.31/0.89 = 0.35 or 35%.

Number needed to treat = 1/Absolute risk reduction = 1/0.31 = 3.2 meaning that in order to benefit one patient we need to treat 3.2 patients.

As a clinical trial progresses, a proportion of subjects may develop the condition of interest, such as the occurrence of carcinoma, or succumb to death, if it is a survival study. To estimate the effect of a hazardous factor on a population, we consider the proportion of the population surviving the hazard and how long individual subjects survive. As different individuals succumb at different time intervals, only the individuals who are not yet affected are at risk at any given time. Already affected subjects, who are removed from the study, no longer have any risk. To statistically quantify the effect of the hazard, the hazard rate and hazard ratio are calculated.

Hazard rate is the proportion of individuals affected by the hazard at a given time divided by the number of individuals who reach that time point without experiencing the hazard. In other words, it is the number of outcomes in a group divided by the number of survivors in that group at a defined instant in time. **Hazard ratio** is the ratio of the hazard rate of the treatment group to the hazard rate of the control or placebo group. It indicates the effectiveness of a treatment in preventing the hazard. A hazard ratio of one means that the hazard is equally affecting both treatment and control groups, and the treatment is not effective in preventing the hazard. While a hazard ratio of less than one indicates that treatment is effective in preventing the hazard, a hazard ratio of greater than one indicates that the treatment is contributing to the hazard (Norman & Streiner, 2009).

Correlation coefficient gives an indication of strength and direction of a linear relationship between two independent continuous variables. Suppose you are curious to know if there is a relationship between body mass index and systolic blood pressure. If so, how strong is this relation and is the relation a positive or a negative one? To answer these questions, we measure the correlation coefficient using the covariance and standard deviation of the two variables (body mass index and systolic blood pressure), which provides a measure of the trend between forecasted values and the clinical trial or real life values. However, it does not provide any clue about the characterization of the values. The correlation coefficient is also known as **Pearson's product moment correlation coefficient** in recognition of the man who first described it. It reveals whether the relation between the two variables is linear, and the extent that each variable deviates from the straight line. The correlation coefficient varies from -1 to +1. A correlation coefficient of zero means that there is no relationship between the two variables, while a correlation coefficient close to 1 indicates that there is a very strong relationship. The positive or negative sign indicates the direction of the relationship.

An important characteristic of a correlation coefficient is that it is free from the units of data and has no dimension. A major limitation of the correlation coefficient is that it is valid only within the range of the data and cannot be applied beyond the data range. Even a strong correlation coefficient (value close to 1 or -1) should not be misinterpreted as implying a **causal relationship** (a change in one variable leading to a change in the other variable). It simply means that both variables are changing together. It is possible that both variables are affected by a third variable, which is causing a change in both variables. For example, a lack of exercise and a high fat diet may be causing both weight gain and an increase in systolic blood pressure. If the data are not normally distributed and the sample collection is not random, or the variable under study is on ordinal scale, **Spearman's rank correlation coefficient** (ρ) should be used.

Regression is a measure of the relationship between a dependent variable, such as a response or an outcome, and an independent variable. The main utility of regression analysis is to use available data in making predictions. For instance, by establishing a regression model, information about immune status, cardiovascular parameters, nutrition status, and bacterial load can be used to make a prediction about the outcome of a patient with an infection. By convention, dependent variables are designated as y and independent variables as x. The independent variable x is used to predict the value of variable y. In regression analysis, one of the parameters has to remain a dependent variable and the other an independent variable; therefore, the two variables cannot be interchanged. The regression analyses are divided into two subgroups of simple linear regression and logistic regression. **Simple linear regression** is conducted when we work with a continuous dependent variable, such as the height of individuals, blood cholesterol level, or oxygen saturation, etc. The simple linear regression is represented by an equation: $\mathbf{y = \alpha + \beta x + \varepsilon,}$ where α is the intercept, β is the slope of the 'line of best fit' representing the relation between variables x and y, and ε is the quantitative difference between observed value Y and the line of regression. If the dependent variable or the independent variable is **dichotomous,** such as infected or not infected, pregnant or not pregnant, cured or not cured, **logistic regression** should be used in the prediction of outcomes. Logistic regression is widely used in clinical research. As an example, consider a study that is conducted to predict the occurrence of heat stroke in males 35-45 years old. The occurrence of heat stroke is influenced by the atmospheric temperature. The predicted probability of heat stroke occurrence is P, whereas $1 - P$ is the probability of non-occurrence. Based on the available data about age and the occurrence of heat stroke, logistic regression can be used to calculate the probability of heat stroke for an individual at a given age.

Survival Analysis deals with the length of time taken by a subject to reach an event. The event could be death or some clinically observable pathological change, such as the development of melanoma. Survival analysis is used to make a prediction about how long a cancer patient survives after receiving a specific medication, or about the average time a group of patients will survive after acquiring HIV. It can also be used to compare the survival time of two groups of patients receiving different treatments. In survival analysis, the effect of a variable on survival of a patient is observed. The subject may be alive at the end of the study, may have died during the course of the study (**censored observations**), or left the study while it was running (**withdrawals**). In survival analysis, it is not necessary for all patients in the study to start at the same time. The key point is the duration of time spent by an individual patient in the study. This flexibility makes this tool very attractive in clinical studies. It helps in determining the effectiveness of a treatment (Belle, Fisher, Heagerty, & Lumley, 2004).

There are many approaches to study survival analysis. The most prominent approach is **Kaplan-Meier survival analysis**. The percentage of surviving subjects is plotted on the y axis, and time is plotted on the x axis (Figure 9.5). The survival curve progresses in vertical steps and horizontal lines. Only survival time and events, such as death, disease occurrence, or reoccurrence, are counted. This approach is used to calculate median survival time (length of time until 50% of the subjects have experienced the event), mean survival time, survival rate at a given time period, and to compare the efficacy of different treatments to alter 'survival.'

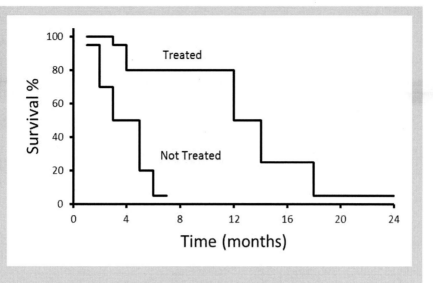

Figure 9.5. Kaplan-Meier Survival Analysis

When to Use Relative Risk, Odds Ratio, and Hazard Ratio?

Relative risks are mostly used in randomized clinical trials, cohort studies, and Poisson regression analysis. Odd ratios are used in case-control studies, retrospective studies, and logistic regression analyses. Hazard ratios are used with survival analyses.

How Distribution of Data Affects the Choice of Statistical Test?

There are certain conditions associated with the use of parametric tests, one of which is that the distribution of data should be normal. Whether or not the data are normally distributed could be determined by a test of 'goodness of fit.' If a population follows a normal distribution, then parametric tests, such as the t-test and ANOVA, could be applied. However, if data distribution is not normal, non-parametric tests, such as Mann-Whitney U test, sign test, Kruskal-Wallis one-way analysis of variance by ranks, and Friedman two-way analysis of variance can be used.

The Appropriate Use of Non-Parametric (e.g., Mann-Whitney U, Wilcoxon) Statistical Tests

When assumptions of normality and homogeneous variance are not met, Mann-Whitney U test and Wilcoxon rank sum test are used to compare two groups. The Mann-Whitney U test is used in place of unpaired t-test to compare two independent groups. It does not require both groups to be of the same size, making it very valuable and handy to use. The data points in both group are given ranks based on magnitude in increasing order, the test statistic is obtained from these ranks, and the hypothesis is tested by comparing the test statistic with a table. The Wilcoxon rank sum test can be used instead of a paired t-test to compare paired groups. It is used when both magnitude and direction of difference (positive or negative) between two paired groups is known, giving it an edge over the sign test, which is limited to magnitude of differences in two paired groups (Portney & Watkins, 2009).

What Is a Confidence Interval?

An interval estimate of a population parameter is more accurate than the single point estimate. Confidence interval helps in making interval estimates about range of population and associated probability of finding the population mean in that range from the sample mean and SD in a normally distributed population. It tells about the lower limit, upper limit, and what is the probability of getting values within that range. For example, in a normal distribution, the interval represented by z value of +1.96 to -1.96 covers 95% of the area. Suppose there is a sample with a mean of 25 and SD 6, then the confidence interval for the sample with 95% probability will be $25\pm (1.96 \times 6)$. The result of the calculations will be 13.24 to 36.76. Based on this, we can conclude that we could be confident that our value of 25 will fall in 13.42 to 36.76 interval 95% of the time. The upper 36.76 and lower 13.42 limits of confidence interval are known as **confidence limits**.

Diagnostic Tests

In ancient times, the identification of disease was heavily based on symptoms. Looking at a patient's condition, a doctor generally attempted to correlate it to a known disease prevalent in that region. With advances in medicine and diagnostic technology, we have much more sophisticated tools to measure certain biomarkers associated with a disease. By comparing the findings with known reference ranges, a more accurate decision can be made about the presence or absence of the disease. Of course, modern-day physicians still rely on symptoms to identify a disorder, but they also have access to diagnostic tests to help in their decision-making.

Diagnostic tests may be used to identify infections, like viral hepatitis, by measuring the level of antibody in blood, or disorders, like cholestasis, by measuring increased plasma levels of enzymes, such as alkaline phosphatase and gamma-glutamyl transpeptidase. The diagnostic tests enable physicians to categorize a patient as positive or negative for the abnormality based on clinical laboratory tests or clinical observations.

The value of a clinical laboratory test lies in its ability to identify a true positive as positive and a true negative as negative. Sensitivity, specificity, and predictive value of the test are characteristics that can be measured to gauge the value of a laboratory test. The clinical **sensitivity** is the ability of a test to identify the patients who are truly positives. The clinical **specificity** is the ability of a test to distinguish those patients who truly do not have the disease. A good test should have high clinical sensitivity and specificity. Clinical sensitivity and specificity are different concepts from analytical sensitivity and specificity. Analytical sensitivity and specificity are concerned with analytical measurement of biomarkers, whereas clinical sensitivity and specificity are concerned with the association of the biomarkers with clinical outcomes or endpoints.

A diagnostic test should help physicians to make correct predictions about the presence or absence of a disease. The ability of a test to make accurate predictions is called **predictive value**. The proportion of true positive observations from a set of observations yielding a positive response in the test is called **positive predictive value**. Similarly, the proportion of true negative results from a set of negative results in a diagnostic test is called **negative predictive value**. Needless to say, clinicians prefer a diagnostic test with high predictive values. Table 9.5 explains clinical sensitivity and specificity.

Table 9.5. Clinical Sensitivity and Specificity

The test	Disease present	No disease
Positive results	60 (a) (True positive)	5 (b) (False positive)
Negative results	30 (c) (False negative)	80 (d) (True Negative)

TP (true positive, have disease), FP (false positive, no disease), FN (false negative, have disease), TN (true negative, no disease).

Sensitivity = a/(a+c) = TP/(TP+FN) = 60/(60+30) = 67%. Therefore, 67% of the time the test can correctly diagnose the patients who have the disease.

Specificity = d/(b+d) = TN/(TN+FP) = 80/(80+5) = 94%. Therefore, 94% of the time the test can correctly identify the individuals who have no disease.

Positive Predictive Value = a/(a+b) = TP/(TP+FP) = 60/(60+5) = 92%. Among those who tested positive, 92% of the time this test correctly identified the individuals who had the disease, whereas 8% of the time this test incorrectly identified healthy individuals as having the disease.

Negative Predictive Value = d/(c+d) = TN/(TN+FN) = 80/(80+30) =73%. Among those who tested negative, 73% of the time the test correctly identified those who had no disease, whereas 27% of the time the test incorrectly identified individuals who had the disease as healthy.

Likelihood ratio positive = sensitivity/(1-specificity) = 0.67/(1-0.94) = 0.67/0.06 = 11.2

Likelihood ratio negative = (1-sensitivity)/specificity = (1-0.67)/0.94 = 0.34/0.94 = 0.36

When comparing different tests to select the best diagnostic test, it is essential to review the clinical sensitivity and specificity of the tests. However, the clinical sensitivity and specificity of a test rely on a cut-off or decision point, which determines the positivity and negativity of the test. Any change in the decision point will change the proportion of positives and negatives, and thus change the sensitivity and specificity of the test. Statisticians have developed **receiver operating characteristic (ROC) curves** as a tool to determine the most medically relevant decision point (DeAngelis, 1990). This is a point where the greatest number of true positives and true negatives will be identified, with tradeoffs depending on the severity of the disease. This graph could relate sensitivity and specificity for any number of cutoffs. The sensitivity (true positives) are graphed on the y axis and 1 - specificity (false positives) are graphed on the x axis (Figures 9.6a and b).

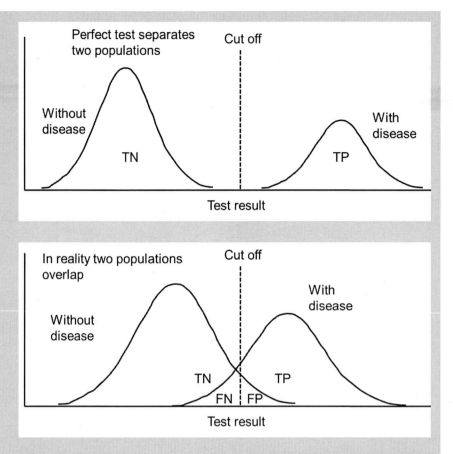

Figures 9.6a & b. Concept of Two Separate Populations With and Without Disease. TN (true negative, no disease), TP (true positive, have disease), FN (false negative, have disease), FP (false positive, no disease).

The position of the cutoff (the clinically relevant decision point) determines the sensitivity, specificity, positive predictive value, and negative predictive value of the test. The cutoff is generally determined from the ROC curve based on the clinical importance of being right (Figure 9.7). There is a tradeoff between sensitivity and specificity.

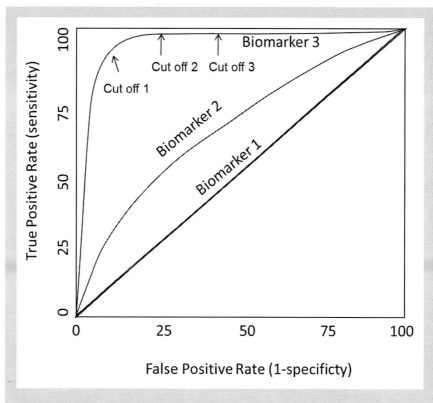

Figure 9.7. ROC Curve

Biomarker 3 has the best clinical sensitivity and specificity as the area under the curve is the greatest for biomarker 3 in comparison to biomarker 1 and biomarker 2. Biomarker 1 has no clinical value. There is no value in choosing cutoff 3 (decision point, marked by arrow) as it provides the same sensitivity as cut off 2, but worse specificity. There is a tradeoff between choosing cutoff 1 versus cutoff 2. For instance, if cut off 2 is chosen, more patients with disease are identified, but then a second more specific test will be needed to identify those who test as false positive.

When a patient visits a doctor's office for a problem, the doctor attempts to make a diagnosis based on symptoms, signs, the duration of problem, normal health parameters, history of the patient, and diagnostic reports. Using information at his/her disposal, the clinician identifies the status of the patient in terms of a **clinical prediction rule** by ascertaining how many criteria are present in the patient. This helps in making a prediction about the possible outcome, and deciding on the best course of treatment. A patient ranked high (meeting many criteria) is more likely to benefit from the designated treatment. A good clinical prediction rule has high sensitivity and specificity, a positive predictive value, and a positive likelihood ratio.

Systematic Review and Meta-Analysis

To utilize the data generated in randomized controlled trials for evidence-based medicine, a literature review of relevant topics is conducted. This is termed as **systematic review** of available literature. Systemic review involves identifying a question, collecting papers and reports that address the question of interest, determining the eligibility of studies based on pre-determined criteria, reviewing results and conclusions of selected studies without bias, identifying the applicable evidence, assimilating the applicable studies to create a 'composite result,' and incorporating the synthesized information in reviews. The major criticism of systematic reviews is that all reviews are not equally reliable (Eyesnck, 1978). In rapidly changing areas of medicine, such as cancer research, systematic reviews become outdated in a year or two. With so many clinical trials being conducted, we can find many studies done on any specific health issue. Different studies involving different sample sizes and subjects yield varied and sometimes opposing results. How do we utilize this varying information to come up with a conclusion that includes aspects of all the studies to obtain a more accurate analysis which can be widely applied to a population? To meet these goals, a meta-analysis is conducted.

Application of statistics on quantitative systematic reviews to get more applicable and accurate findings is called **meta-analysis**. This method was developed by Gene V. Glass in the 1970s and involves standardizing and normalizing different studies to get a summary (from a few to hundreds of studies). It involves deciding the topic of study, identifying relevant studies, and determining the eligibility of studies. Results are obtained from the eligible studies, and an effect size statistic is calculated from quantitative observations obtained from pooled studies of varying sample size, involving different methods of interpretation. Observations are appropriately standardized and compared. **Meta-analysis** enjoys many advantages over **systematic review** as it provides findings with greater statistical power that can be generalized and applied to a study population with a high confidence level (Lipsey & Wilson, 2001). Usually, meta-analysis relative measures, like odd ratios or relative risk, are used as these remain nearly the same across the studies. The standardized difference is taken while comparing the continuous variable. Meta-analysis suffers from several disadvantages. Different quantitative variables are coded to get a widely applicable outcome. In addition, the meta-analysis is not sensitive to biological relevance of a variable, and even though statistically robust, some variables may not have any clinical context or 'practical' effect. The research questions being investigated may not be the same in all studies. Most of the time overlapping questions are included. Meta-analysis involves quantitative comparison, while in some studies qualitative variables are also critical. Hence, a good strategy to effectively summarize studies is to conduct both a systematic review and a meta-analysis. In order to generate a high quality meta-analysis, it is imperative that only standard and flawless studies be included. It is difficult to find studies that are considered high quality by everyone. Nonetheless, with its benefits overweighing the drawbacks, the meta-analysis is a very effective tool in generating and acquiring the essence of the best findings (Slavin, 1986).

Statistical software:

List of statistical packages: http://en.wikipedia.org/wiki/List_of_statistical_packages

SPSS: http://www.spss.com/

GraphPad: http://www.graphpad.com/welcome.htm

Useful online websites:

For a 2x2 Contingency Table:
http://faculty.vassar.edu/lowry/odds2x2.html

Risk Reduction Calculator:
http://araw.mede.uic.edu/cgi-bin/nntcalc.pl

Roc curve: http://www.medcalc.be/manual/roc.php

Chi Square test: http://www.xmarks.com/site/people.ku.edu/~preacher/chisq/chisq.htm

Chi Square test:
http://math.hws.edu/javamath/ryan/ChiSquare.html

For the difference between odds ratio and relative risk see: http://en.wikipedia.org/wiki/Relative_risk

For hazard ratio see: http://en.wikipedia.org/wiki/Hazard_ratio

For sample size and power of analysis: http://www.stat.ubc.ca/~rollin/stats/ssize/

For one-tailed and two-tailed test: http://www.ats.ucla.edu/stat/mult_pkg/faq/general/tail_tests.htm

A guide for the use of statistical tests

Short lists of statistical tests which can be used in clinical studies are indicated in the following three tables.

Table 9.6: Selecting an appropriate test (quantitative variable for parametric data).

Conditions	Test
One group, parametric	One sample t-test
Two groups, parametric, unpaired	Two sample t-test
Two groups, parametric, paired	Paired t-test
More than two groups, parametric, unpaired	One-way ANOVA
More than two groups, parametric, related	ANOVA

Table 9.7: Selecting an appropriate test (quantitative variable for non-parametric data).

Conditions	Test
One group, Non-parametric	Sign test
Two groups, non-parametric, unpaired	Wilcoxon rank sum test
Two groups, non-parametric, paired	Sign test, Wilcoxon signed rank test
More than two groups, non-parametric, unpaired	Kruskal Wallis one-way ANOVA
More than two groups, non-parametric, related	Friedman two-way ANOVA

Table 9.8: Selecting an appropriate test (nominal variable).

Conditions	Test
One group	Test of single proportion
Two groups, assumptions allowed, unpaired	Chi-square test
Two groups, assumptions not allowed, unpaired	Fisher's exact test
Two groups, paired	McNemar's test
More than two groups, assumptions allowed, independent	Chi-square test
More than two groups, assumptions not allowed, independent	Combine groups Chi-squared test

10 | Data Fraud and Authorship

Vinod K. Sethi, MD

Scientists in the field of biomedical research carry an important role in the development of newer techniques, devices, and drugs for the betterment of the society. The public has tremendous respect for the scientific community as such. The Oxford dictionary describes the scientist as a person who is studying or has expert knowledge of one or more physical sciences. The research community has "zero tolerance" toward scientific fraud, especially in the medical field. Legally speaking, scientific fraud is a deliberate misrepresentation by someone who knows the truth (Pryor, Habermann, & Broome, 2007; Federal Register, 2005).

The Department of Health and Human Services defines scientific misconduct as, "Misconduct means fabrication, falsification, or plagiarism in proposing or performing research funded by the National Science Foundation (NSF), reviewing research proposals submitted to NSF, or in reporting research results funded by NSF."

- 45 C.F.R. s 689.1. Fabrication means making up data or results and recording or reporting them.

- 45 C.F.R. §689.1. Falsification means manipulating research materials, equipment, or processes, or changing or omitting data or results such that the research is not accurately represented in the research record.
- 45 C.F.R. §689.1. Plagiarism means the appropriation of another person's ideas, processes or words without giving appropriate credit.

Characteristics of research misconduct include not following the accepted practices/methods of research, must be committed knowingly or recklessly, and allegations must be proved by preponderance of the evidence (42 Code of Federal Regulations Part 93.104). It does not include honest errors.

Although these definitions of misconduct strictly apply to the research funded by the different agencies of the Department of Health and Human Services, many private trusts and other agencies stipulate that the same standards be followed. The incidence of misconduct is not very well known. In a commentary on "Scientists Behaving Badly," Martinson, Anderson, and de Vries stated, "U.S. scientists engage in a range of behaviors extending far beyond falsification, fabrication, and plagiarism" (Martinson, Anderson, & de Vries, 2005). Based on a survey sent to over 7,000 scientists working in the U.S. and receiving grants from the National Institutes of Health, the incidence of misconduct with falsification, fabrication, and plagiarism is less than 2%, but out of these one in three admitted to committing one of these behaviors: falsifying or 'cooking' research data, ignoring major aspects of human-subject requirements, not properly disclosing involvement in firms whose products are based on one's own research, overlooking others' use of flawed data or questionable interpretation of data, changing the design, methodology, or results of a study in response to pressure from a funding source, dropping observations or data points from analyses based on a gut feeling that they were inaccurate, and some others. For more details, see Martinson, Anderson, & deVries, 2005.

Pryor and associates conducted a nation-wide survey of research supervisors. Out of 5,302 surveys sent, 1,645 responded. Amongst the responders, 18% reported first-hand knowledge of research misconduct (Pryor, Habermann, & Broome, 2007). This was commonly reported from academic medical centers. Perceived prevalence of plagiarism was 0.2%, falsifying data 0.5%, intentional protocol violations 1.2%, coercion of potential subjects 1.2%, deliberate double billing for study 0.6%, selective dropping out of data from outlier cases 0.7%, falsification of bio sketch 0.1%, resume reference list 0.1%, disagreement about authorship 1.5%, and pressure from study sponsor 0.3%. In a meta-analysis of 21 surveys, Fanelli reported that a pooled weighted average of 1.97% (N=7, 95% CI: 0.86-4.45) of scientists admitted to having fabricated, falsified, or modified data or results at least once – a serious form of misconduct by any standard – and up to 33.7% admitted other questionable research practices. In surveys asking about the behavior of colleagues, admission rates were 14.12% (N=12; 95% CI: 9.91-19.72) for falsification, and up to 72% for other questionable research practices (Fanelli, 2009).

The U.S. constitution has created a unique system of checks and balances whereby the free press plays an important role in keeping the balance in our society. A joint poll conducted by the Office of Research Integrity and the Gallop Company reported that there are more suspected cases of misconduct in research than are reported to the appropriate authorities (Steneck, 2011). Cases of misconduct are not limited to research in the public sector alone. Gardner, Lidz, and Harwing reviewed a survey based on published authors of pharmaceutical trials that found 17% of the respondents had knowledge of misrepresentation of fabricated data, compared to 0.3% of federally funded U.S. researchers self-reporting falsifying the data (Gardner, Litz, & Hartwig, 2005).

What are the reasons scientists engage in activities that are not conducive to expected behavior? The pressures from many academic institutions to engage in research and publish are among the requirements for promotion. Peer recognition and positions in professional associations are other factors. Most of the data reported in the literature are based on the surveys conducted. Only one study done by Davis, Riske-Morris, and Diaz studied the closed case files from the Office of Research Integrity (ORI) (Davis, Riske-Morris, & Diaz, 2007). Based on the 104 files reviewed, they reported seven clusters that were mentioned by the scientists being investigated.

Plagiarism, falsification, fabrication, and combinations of these were common types of misconduct. Reasons described by the scientists being investigated were clustered in seven groups:

- Personal and professional stressors
- Organizational climate factors
- Job insecurities
- Rationalization A: A lack of control over one's environment, jumping the gun to disseminate findings, and lying in order to preserve the truth.
- Personnel inhibitions
- Rationalization B: Difficult job and task frustrations
- Personality factors

Pressure from the academic institution to perform for the purpose of promotion was a common reason mentioned. In addition to this, environment of the institution and job insecurity were also reasons given. This study, however, is based only on the subjects who were investigated and reprimanded by ORI. It does not include the data on subjects being investigated and not found guilty of misconduct. Data fraud is very difficult to detect. The incidence of this problem is unknown. Based on a survey, the authors of every fourth primary research paper published in the *Journal of American Medical Association* (2001-2003), *Canadian Medical Association* (2001-2003), *British Medical Journal* (1998-2000), and *Lancet* (1998-2000) reported that 94% of the authors accepted the full responsibility for the integrity of the data, 21% discovered that the data published previously and co-authored were incorrect (Baerlocher, O'Brien, Newton, Gautam, & Noble, 2010). Twenty-one percent had encountered a disagreement on the data amongst different co-authors, and they withdrew their name from the authorship. Four percent of the authors admitted that their previous published work had fraudulent data. Nearly ten percent did not use safeguards for data collection.

In spite of this and other data, only 201 cases were reported to ORI in 2008. Of the 201 allegations made to ORI (or to NIH and reported to ORI) in 2008, 52 were assessed by ORI in detail for a potential inquiry or investigation; five of the assessments were opened as cases in 2008. Of the remaining Pre-Inquiry Assessments, 12 were administratively closed after being reviewed, and 35 remained open at the end of the year (ORI, 2008). Comparing the data from surveys with the reported cases, it seems that many cases were not reported.

Gross described the safeguards for a well-designed study as (1) pre-determine the patient selection method, (2) specify the causal or protective agent at the outset, (3) provide for unbiased data collection, (4) avoid differences in patient recall of past events, (5) avoid constrained selection of cases and controls, (6) use similar diagnostic tests, (7) use the same case finding methods, (8) use the same demographic criteria, (9) use population with similar risk factors, (10) assure that the patient is not inadvertently using the study agent before the diagnosis is made, and (11) assure that patients exposed to the study agent have an equal chance of inclusion in the groups, whether or not they are ill (Gross, 1984). These safeguards should be used in data collection, and analytical methods should be used to analyze the data.

Who Can Do It?

In the research studies, a number of personnel are usually involved, including a principal investigator, co-investigator, clinical research nurse, lab technicians, data-collectors (electronic or otherwise), data analyst, study coordinators, administrative staff, and even the subjects themselves. Honest errors can occur at each level; however, there is a potential for fraud at all stages of research. Joint studies done at different research centers may have many issues on the data being reported. The ORI defines "fabrication" of data as "making up data or results and recording or reporting them" (Steneck, 2011). Falsification of data might be in proposing, designing, performing, recording, supervising or reviewing research, or in reporting research results. Falsification also includes acts of omission and commission.

Definition from FDA: Falsification and or fabrication are done in a number of ways. Wollen and Hage from the section of "Good Clinical Practices Branch" of the FDA, describe multiple examples of these (Wollen & Hage, 2001). Substituting EKGs, misrepresentation of dates, duplicate X-rays with different names, blank lab reports to fill-in, using fake subjects (obituary names), testing done after the subjects died, same subject different names, non-existent subjects created, dates changed in records to match wash-out periods, consent not signed before entering the study, unqualified staff doing physical examination, inadequate records, failure to report changes in research, bogus lab results reported, changing the source document, sample study-wide from only a few subjects, subjects received prohibited medication while on study, and failure to report adverse events.

Misconduct in plagiarism involves using other people's ideas, words or processes without giving proper credit. Office of Scientific Integrity has the details on rules of plagiarism (ORI, 2009; ORI, 2010a). Most of the problem lies with authorship issues of scientific publications. Copying of paragraphs or phrases falls in this category.

Methods of Detecting Falsification and Fabrication

It is a difficult and time-consuming task to detect falsification and fabrication. Research misconduct can be revealed by statistical analysis of data submitted in research publications. For more information, refer to a chapter written by Stephen Evans on "Can statistical analysis reveal research misconduct?" in the book *On Fraud and Misconduct* by Wells and Farthing (2008). Evans describes the details and detection of data, whether it is genuine, altered, or invented. Use of different analytical methods may be a problem. Jaffer and Cameron (2006) opined that it is easier to detect falsification in multicenter trial studies.

Plagiarism

As described earlier, plagiarism is defined by the NIH as the appropriation of another person's ideas, processes, or words without giving appropriate credit. The issues related to this problem happen in the area of authorship. Claxton wrote an excellent review on this subject (Claxton, 2005). Conflict of interest while interpreting the data can be an area worth looking into.

Many research studies specially funded by non-NIH grants may have a bias in the mind of a researcher during the process of data analysis or writing up the research report for publication. In an article for publication done by multiple authors, the question about the first author, second author, and last author may be difficult to resolve. Naming a superior as an author who has not contributed to the research and has not participated in writing up the paper can be a problem. So called "Honorary Authorship" is not looked upon as standard practice. By the same token, not giving authorship to people who were involved with the research project will qualify as plagiarism. Sometimes two authors will give authorship to each other in research they have conducted independently. In research conducted at multiple centers, it may be difficult to prove honorary authorship. Cases have been described in the literature where an organization conducted and wrote up a research project, and gave credit to a prominent writer or scientist just for reviewing and signing off on it. This is a deplorable act and must be condemned. Many times, the same article is published in more than one journal under different names, but with the same research data. Many journals are asking the writers to sign a document that this has not happened before they even consider the article for publication. However, if the data being reported in the second article has not been published, although it is a part of the same research, it is permissible. There are professional writers who will write up the articles once they are provided with the data. This is another reason for concern. NIH has delineated the issues on authorship (NIH, 2008). Hoen et al. have discussed the issue of authorship order (Hoen, Walvoort, & Overbeke, 1998). IRBs of the different academic centers and the various journals may have their own rules for publication. The International Committee of Medical Journal Editors states that "authorship credit should be based on: 1) substantial contributions to conception and design, acquisition of data, or analysis and interpretation of data; 2) drafting the article or revising it critically for important intellectual content; and 3) final approval of the version to be published. Authors should meet conditions one, two, and three." The rest of the contributors can be mentioned in Acknowledgements (ICMJE, 2009).

Reporting

Anyone can report to the IRB of the institution where the research is being done. The people who report fraud are usually members of the research team, such as research technicians, clinical research nurses, data analysts, or one of the co-investigators who has withdrawn his or her name from the research or publication. It is extremely important that they are protected from repercussions. By regulation, each extramural entity that applies for a biomedical or behavioral research, research-training, or research-related grant or cooperative agreement under the Public Health Service (PHS) Act must establish policies and procedures that provide for "undertaking diligent efforts to protect the positions and reputations of those persons who, in good faith, make allegations" (42 C.F.R. Part 50.103(d)(13); ORI, 1995). The institutions do not have to follow exactly the guidelines set by the Commission on Research Integrity so long as they have procedures set to meet the regulatory requirements. The regulations call for protection of the whistle-blowers who make allegations in good faith. It is the responsibility of the institutions to protect the whistleblowers. Gunsalus and Rennie (2008) have reviewed this subject. There are three ways the whistle-blower can report the alleged misconduct: to a person in charge at the institution, to the ORI, or directly to the Office of the United States Congress. Whistle-blowing, however, is sometimes not without consequences. Kesselheim et al. studied 26 whistle-blowers and found that 82% reported facing pressures from the companies they were working for (Kesselheim, Studdert, & Mello, 2010). In eight cases, financial hardships were reported, and six reported family conflicts leading to divorces, severe marital strain, or other family conflicts. Thirteen out of 26 faced various health issues. However, 22 out of 26 claimed that they had become whistle-blowers for ethical, psychological, or religious reasons.

Consequences of Misconduct

Once the misconduct is proven, the ORI may impose the following (ORI, 2010b):

- Debarment from eligibility to receive Federal funds for grants and contracts

- Prohibition from service on PHS advisory committees, peer review committees, or as consultants

- Certification of information sources by respondent that is forwarded by institution

- Certification of data by institution
- Imposition of supervision on the respondent by the institution
- Submission of a correction of a published article by respondent
- Submission of a retraction of a published article by respondent

Usually, the actions are in effect from one to three years; however, life-time durations have been imposed in some cases. In addition, the institution where the scientist is working may have additional rules for dealing with misconduct. The officer in charge of the institution may decide to notify law enforcement agencies, professional societies, licensing boards, co-investigators, journals where the research article may have been published, the whistle-blower, if any was involved, and the agencies responsible for funding or sponsoring the research project.

Prevention of Fraud and Misconduct

The cost of misconduct to the institution and the individual involved is beyond the monetary value. The reputation of the laboratory involved and institutional prestige is at stake. Loss of future funding from the sponsoring agencies could be devastating for the institution. Michalek et al. have estimated the cost of one investigation itself to be $525,000 (Michalek, Hutson, Wicher, & Trump, 2010). Besides the costs to the institution, no one can estimate the cost of published research and its impact on the citations it has received, effect on research being done based on the research in question, and its impact on public health. The cost of the consequences to the scientist in question is far reaching. It is prudent, therefore, that we take steps to prevent the problem of misconduct in research. Undergraduate and postgraduate education and educating the faculty through faculty development courses are some of the measures institutions can take. The role of the IRBs in granting permission to do research is extremely important. Research conduct training through organizations, such as the Collaborative Institutional Training Initiative (CITI), is usually a requirement before the IRB allows research personnel to take part in an approved project (NIH, 2010).

11 | Advice on Writing a Research Grant

Candace A. Myers, PhD

Funding is not always a problem. If you have the time and do the work yourself, case reports and retrospective chart reviews can be completed without a budget. Low cost research can also be conducted if you have access to a database, propose an observational study, and analyze the data on your own time. Studies that involve surveys may cost little or nothing if your institution subscribes to an online survey service or you write and distribute your survey on your own. You will probably need the help of a statistician, but many institutions have statisticians available to assist investigators. The other forms of clinical research are usually quite expensive. The researcher must pay the salaries of highly skilled personnel to perform the work, and for costly laboratory tests or procedures. This brings us to our topic of **grant writing**. The topic is well represented on the Internet and numerous experts offer workshops

The most important step in securing funding is to define a worthwhile and realistic project. Each proposal should be significant and unique. You should present a novel and interesting idea that addresses an important and timely problem. You will need to clearly define your idea and logically convey your plans for the research. Explain how your ability, the resources available at your institution, and the skills and experience of the scientists involved in your project are sufficient to accomplish your goals. The amount of funding you request should be sensible and well justified.

Your Idea

The questions you want to answer with your research must be compelling, original, and significant. Identify a specific problem worth answering. You must have a clear concept of your goal and identify the means to achieve it. In formulating your idea, you must think within the constraints of the funding period and the funds available from the organization that you have identified as a potential benefactor for your research expenses. Conduct a thorough literature search and collect relevant citations to support your contentions. You will need to demonstrate that your work is novel because few organizations will want to spend their funds to repeat work that has already been published. The background work you do to become fully aware of the literature will pay off by improving your research question, as well as being useful when you write the background and rationale section of your application. You will need to explain what is known, why it is important to learn more, and what an advancement in your area of interest could produce.

Seek the advice of your colleagues and mentors. Do they agree that the topic of your project needs to be addressed? This is the time to refine your idea and look for the most promising paths toward achieving your goal. You also need to consider your skill set and your ability to devote the time needed to attain the goal. You will need to convince the application reviewers that you have the expertise and the time to conduct the research. Candidly consider your situation and ensure that you don't set yourself up for failure by overextending yourself or exaggerating your abilities. Reviewers will reject projects if they think the proposal is too ambitious for the time and money you specify.

General Rules for Writing

As a general rule, avoid very long or short paragraphs. Reviewers, tired from reading applications, will be turned-off by a page-long paragraph and annoyed by choppy one-sentence-long paragraphs. Avoid clichés and do not add empty generalities that sound good, but do not say anything. Keep your sentences relatively short and declarative. If you cannot read the sentence aloud without taking a breath, the sentence is too long. Restrict your use of underlining, capitalizations, italics, and bolding. A little can be very effective, but overuse can be irritating to the reader and counterproductive. Minimize the use of acronyms and abbreviations, and ALWAYS define them the first time they are used. Few things are more irritating to a reader than having to scan previous pages to be reminded of what EJBC stands for. Only rely on abbreviations and acronyms for phrases that are used frequently (more than three or four times in the span of a couple of paragraphs). Be positive about your work, and do not use words that convey doubt. Substitute the words expect or will for words like hope, try, may, believe, or could. You will conduct the research with the reasonable expectation of your described outcome. Choose your words carefully and check your spelling. If you submit an application on paper, use a font size that the reviewer can read without straining. Usually a ten-point font should be your limit, and remember that the writing on your graphics needs to be large enough to read.

Identify a Potential Funding Source

The next step is to identify a likely funding agency, foundation, or organization with a mission that your research will help achieve. Spend some time on their website reviewing the funding organization's mission statement, former supported projects, and their stated areas of emphasis for the current round of support. If your project does not meet these requirements, your application will be tossed at the first round and may never even be read. Some organizations provide the name and contact information for an advisor at the agency who can answer questions and provide guidance to potential applicants. They will know what their agency is looking for and can offer valuable advice. Keep looking until you find a funding source that is a good match for your project. If your project is relevant to their goals, you will want to emphasize that relevance when you describe your research.

Types of funding sources were described in Chapter 12. They all have specific application processes, and these instructions must be followed to the letter. There are usually strict deadlines. Most applications are submitted online. Proposals that are too long, late, or even typed in the wrong font are culled from the stack of submissions and never even considered. Follow the instructions EXACTLY.

Some organizations require a one or two page letter of intent that describes your planned work. If the funding organization is impressed by your letter of intent, you will be invited to submit a full application. If your letter of intent is rejected, you and the funding agency will have been saved a lot of work.

Grant Request Components

Grant applications are usually divided into sections and limited in length. If you have the space, use sub-headings to help clarify the intent of each section. Throughout your application, be succinct and well organized. Keep the focus of the funding agency in mind and make the 'fit' between your project and the goals of the agency crystal clear. Most applications include the following sections:

- Overview/Executive Summary/Objectives
- Background and Rationale
- Personnel
- Experimental Design and Methods
- Budget and Budget Justification
- Timetable
- Outcomes and Limitations

Overview/Executive Summary/Objectives

A well-written overview or executive summary is of key importance to a successful application. Ideally, this one page document will be easy to read and understood by any intelligent reader. This short document will either draw the reader in and set them up to be an advocate for the project, or turn them off so that they perceive the task of reviewing the application as an arduous assignment. The overview will summarize the entire proposal and serve as a blueprint for the full project.

The overview/executive summary may be called by different names in different application formats. It could be called the specific aims page, the significance and rationale, the pre-proposal, or the letter of intent. Regardless, the overview/executive summary requires a significant effort by the author and input from colleagues willing to provide constructive criticism. Like an abstract for a scientific article, this is most easily compiled after the full application has been written. Write it after you have thoroughly answered all the other sections of the proposal. Go back and summarize the proposal. If a good flow in the overview is lacking, you may need to review the entire proposal to ensure that linkages between the various sections of the proposal make sense to the reader.

Describe the goal of your research and what steps you plan to take to achieve this goal. An over-riding objective is often sub-divided into a small number of specific aims. Briefly describe each goal, list the planned studies or activities to accomplish the goal, and explain the expected outcomes.

Background/Needs Assessment/Rationale

Introduce the problem that the research project will address. Provide a historical prospective. As you develop this section of the application, you need to thoroughly cover what is known and where the gaps and limitations in the current knowledge lie. The background is the base upon which you will build your justification for conducting the research project you seek to fund. You will end by describing a critical need to fund the present project. You will want to close this section with a discussion of how the success of your project will impact the field, such as lead to the discovery of new drugs or improve the understanding of the pathogenic process. You may be asked to describe the economic impact of your discoveries.

Cite credible literature sources to substantiate every assertion made. If you provide a description of the size of the problem or prevalence of the disease, cite a reliable, recent source for the information. Cite original research. You may read review articles to locate original research documents, but do not list a review article as the source for an argument that should be supported by original research. Go back to the original article, read it, and ensure that it actually supports the claim you are making. Make sure that each of your citations is complete and absolutely correct.

Within this section, you will need to describe your preliminary studies. This section establishes the feasibility that the research you are proposing will be successfully executed. Previous work will demonstrate your competence and experience in the field. It should never contain work that others have done unless they are collaborators on your project. The preliminary data should directly support the projected studies, and each piece should lead the reviewer to the next study with an understanding of why the work was done and what was achieved. The preliminary studies should outline the incremental accomplishments of the investigators, and culminate with the clear justification for the proposed study. Focus on the results that indicate that the proposed work will probably succeed.

Accumulating preliminary data is typically a challenge for young investigators. Ideally, you learned techniques and obtained some experience while working with a funded mentor. You might seek departmental or institutional funding to conduct a pilot study or to gather the preliminary data needed for a grant application.

Mention your ethical considerations in conducting the research. Explain that if funded you will obtain approval for the study from your local Institutional Review Board (IRB). You will minimize risks to subjects and satisfy all regulatory concerns. Most grants are approved with the contingency that approval from the local IRB will be obtained before the funds are delivered.

Personnel and Environment

Most grant applications require information about the experience and capabilities of the principal investigator and any senior or key personnel. This is where you will document the qualifications of the applicants, coworkers, and collaborators. The reviewer must be convinced that the investigator has the appropriate credentials to successfully execute the proposed project. NIH has a biographical sketch format that is often requested by funding sources, but some foundations ask for a copy of each person's curriculum vitae (CV). Refer to the specific instructions for each application. The biosketch represents an opportunity for the applicant to strategically present up-to-date and maximally supportive information about the research team.

A new applicant is not likely to have a great deal of information to include on a biosketch or CV. Resist the inclination to pad the biosketch or include questionable accolades/achievements. You may include the name of the applicant's doctoral and/or postdoctoral mentor and the title of a dissertation in the bibliography section. As a courtesy, provide to reviewers (as an appendix) an abstract of the dissertation and copies of any submitted or accepted manuscripts that would be difficult for the reviewer to obtain.

Reviewers are also concerned about the environment and the resources available to the applicant. Among the important resources of concern to reviewers is the intellectual environment of your institution. Will the work be conducted in proximity to other funded applicants who make for a scholarly work environment? Data on previous awards to the institution and institutional support for research may be supplied. A catalog of essential equipment and services that are available to the investigator are also important. An expectation exists that a qualified applicant will already have access to a majority of the equipment required.

Experimental Design and Methods

The experimental design and methods is a crucial section of a grant application. The experimental design must be sufficient to answer the questions posed by the project. Although not as detailed as a clinical protocol, the methods must describe exactly how you plan to achieve your research objectives. The applicant must provide enough information for the reviewer to critically evaluate the project. Describe where the study will be conducted and the availability of laboratory space, equipment, analytical tools, or services. Describe the population, distribution of ethnic groups, races, age groups, and socioeconomic classes of potential subjects. For clinical trials, describe how subjects will be recruited and how the sample size was determined. What randomization procedures will be employed?

How will samples be collected, stored, transported, and analyzed? Laboratory techniques should be described in sufficient detail to prove that valid methodology exists and that success is feasible within the hands of the applicant. Data management, protection, and analysis should be described and statistical methods outlined.

Budget and Budget Justification

The amount of financial support requested in the grant application is dictated by the proposal. If you ask for too much or too little, you will lose credibility in the eyes of the reviewer. Carefully review the funding agency's instructions. Some grants do not allow funds to be spent for certain purposes. An otherwise excellent application can be rejected because of an oversight in this section.

Direct Costs

Personnel salary support usually represents the most costly subsection of the budget. Carefully analyze what each member of the study team will do for the project and estimate a percentage of each person's full-time work time that will be committed to the project. Multiply the worker's salary by the percent time commitment to determine the salary support to request for each team member. Fringe benefits are the expenses beyond salaries, borne by the institution for each employee. They include health benefits, leave time, and retirement benefits and are different for each employee, depending on their individual benefits package. The Office of Sponsored Programs or Human Resources Department at your institution will help you estimate each study member's fringe benefits. Fringe benefits to charge to the research budget are calculated for each member of the study team in accord with their time commitments to the project.

Equipment requests are often allowed by granting agencies, but it is generally advisable to limit your requests for expensive equipment. Reviewers often see it as the institution's responsibility to supply the core equipment needed for research and are not inclined to purchase an expensive piece of equipment that will outlast the length of the project. Expendable supplies and reagents are usually required to conduct a project. It is important to consider every aspect of the study and develop a supply list sufficient to cover all proposed activities. Other costs to consider are travel expenses for collaborations or scientific meetings, publication expenses, stipends for subjects, study drugs, and clinical chemistry costs. Cost account all proposed supplies and services based on actual invoices or catalog prices. For multi-year projects, conservatively calculate an inflation rate for subsequent years (two to four percent annually).

Indirect Costs

Indirect costs are probably the most important budgetary item for the sponsoring institution. These are the facilities and administrative costs over and above the direct costs required to actually accomplish the research study. Indirect costs are awarded to the institution to provide for the infrastructure that allows research to be undertaken. Heat, electricity, water, sewage, and janitorial services fall into this category, along with the actual roof over the researchers' heads. For federally-funded projects, indirect rates can be 25% to 50%. Most private foundations allow less, and some funding agencies are unwilling to pay any indirect costs. Again, it is the responsibility of the applicant to determine the policy of the targeted funding agency and ascertain the institution's willingness to submit a grant application under certain conditions.

Many grant opportunities publish a funding limit. This limit should be considered in terms of realistically envisioning the scope of the proposed research project. Applicants are contracting to produce an estimated amount of work product for a particular cost. The application will include sections to justify the expenses and explain how the funds will be spent to reach the study objectives. In formulating the budget, request funds sufficient to perform the proposed work and credibly justify each expense.

Timetable

This need not be an elaborate description of the study, but it should be a reality check for the applicant. Considering the personnel time allotted, the availability of subjects, the time needed for analyses, and the many, many other time constraints, develop a reasonable schedule for accomplishing the project's objectives. This might be presented as a table with monthly or quarterly blocks representing the various study activities.

Outcomes and Limitations of the Proposed Research

An applicant may be asked to describe the possible limitations of his/her study design. A reviewer could envision the obstacles to success as too great and reject the proposal. Therefore, it is important for the applicant to address any limitation to their approach and to let the reviewers know they are aware of potential problems and have alternative strategies to employ if they encounter them.

There may be an opportunity to describe the strengths of the project and the contributions that will be realized if the project is funded and successful.

References

References should be cited at the end of each of the sentences where some claim is made in your background and methods section using a superscript. Citations are numbered in the order they appear in the text. The bibliography should be organized in the same manner and should follow an accepted standard style. If none is specified, use the American Medical Association's Manual of Style (http:// healthlinks.washington.edu/hsl/styleguides/ama.html).

Revision - Revision - Revision

Obtaining constructive criticism from team members is a no-brainer. Study team members will be motivated to submit the best application possible. Obtaining the honest and thorough criticism from a knowledgeable colleague is a greater challenge. In order to meet application deadlines, this means that the applicant must factor time for review and revision into the application preparation schedule. Experienced investigators plan ahead and allow time for this step. They also solicit meaningful, albeit at times painful, constructive criticism from colleagues they can trust with their innovative research ideas. These colleagues must be willing to take the time to thoroughly review the draft. A cursory examination and a flattering assessment are of no help to the applicant.

What if the Application is Rejected

Unfortunately, most grant applications are not funded. If rejected, try to obtain the reviewers comments and any scoring information. Thoughtfully consider the reviewers' comments. If the reviewers identified legitimate weaknesses in the proposal, revise the project, and resubmit it in the next funding cycle. If they suggested additional pilot work, try to find a way to beef-up your preliminary data. If the reviewers misunderstood some aspect of the proposal, do a better job explaining your intent in the next revision. Don't give up. Each revision can improve the application. Resubmit to the same organization or to a different foundation or agency.

12 | The NIH Scientific Review and Ten Commandments for Grant Success

Golder N. Wilson, MD, PhD

The National Institutes of Health (NIH) is probably the most prestigious source for grant support. Emphasis in this chapter is on pre-submission thinking about NIH grant applications to help the new investigator understand the NIH review process, so the considerable time needed for grant submission is not wasted on malformed applications.

The Nature of Basic and Translational Research

The philosopher Michel Foucault (1994) retraced the change in medical "gaze" as physicians went from patients to their tissues and cells. He recognized that the first step was in abstracting the disease from the patient, distinguishing necessary from fortuitous (individual, circumstantial) symptoms. Then the disease essence, inferred by observation of commonalities in diverse affected patients, was accorded to properties of tissues and cells, from the ragged red fibers of muscles with defective mitochondria to the delta F-508 mutation in cystic fibrosis. This transformation from signs and symptoms, such as the white ash-leaf spot of tuberous sclerosis to its imaged cardiac tumors and two genetic loci, was tremendously powerful. The biologic relationships unraveled by basic science could be applied to human disease: cells have metabolism, compartments, constituents of lipid, protein, and nucleic acid; the zygote transforms to organism through growth, differentiation, pattern formation; and organisms are guided by their gene set (genome), modified by epigenesis to produce RNA (transcriptome) and protein (proteome) sets that account for tissue structure and function. The result was a profusion of laboratory techniques that paralleled clinical observation and a gap, even a tension, between the disease defined by molecular traits and its expression in each individual, the age-old difference between reductionist science and the human soul.

The result of what might be called the biologic revolution as it affects medicine is that any physician wishing to compete in translation or application of basic science must acquire training and sophistication in these techniques. For success, the physician must either develop sufficient skill to perform and supervise experiments or sufficient understanding to collaborate in a meaningful way with those who have laboratory expertise. An important aspect of this training is to appreciate the enormous time requirements for laboratory work. Like molecules of a gas, laboratory work can expand to occupy any available scheduling space. In addition, productive researchers need uninterrupted time to concentrate while in the laboratory. This reality puts the physician-researcher in a quandary. How will you handle that telephone call in the middle of an experiment, a defining moment for any physician-researcher? You can either dodge the call or put down the pipette, choosing between patient and experiment. Laboratory training is not only technical, it also teaches a physician-researcher how to handle scheduling conflicts and, over time, will help you determine whether you prefer patients or protocols.

Another key lesson of research training relates to your ability to develop skills: it is one thing to master subject matter and techniques, but can you be a good investigator? (See commandment one.) The latter ability requires envisioning a sequence of logical steps that will dissect a problem and includes familiarity with successful approaches from the literature, an innate ability for problem-solving, a focus on one experimental path, while avoiding many detours, and leadership, since you will need at least one technician and preferably students to accomplish significant amounts of lab work. The ability to see connections between diverse phenomena, so critical to clinical diagnosis, may be a handicap for basic research. For clinicians already balancing multiple roles and multiple activities, multiple projects will usually be a death-knell for achieving competitive funding.

The successful grant applicant will have the investigator's ability to focus on a single project and to conceptualize a single path, resisting detours offered by new techniques. Again I would emphasize that the most important parts of an NIH grant are its preliminary thinking and preliminary results. I have heard several successful grant recipients opine that they had fulfilled most of the grant protocol by the time it was funded.

The nature of basic science as it relates to medicine, then, is to:

- Formulate relationships based on observation
- Translate clinical phenomena into those measured by instruments
- Deduce which step-wise approaches are likely to yield definitive results

A brilliant example of this process resulted in Texas' first Nobel Prize (Goldstein & Brown, 2009). Brown and Goldstein made the clinical observation that heart attacks arise from many factors. In order to formulate a study to identify the important ones, they focused on unusual heart attacks in young people, and translated the young victims' susceptibility to heart disease into cells with poor uptake of cholesterol. They followed this clue like a laser from receptor protein to its gene, from altered exon sequence in familial hypercholesterolemia to milder disease from alterations in upstream regulatory elements. Through a medical genetics fellowship and post-doctoral training, Brown and Goldstein learned a repertoire of techniques, applied them to focused investigations, and followed their stepwise application to a new molecular basis for heart disease. Brown and Goldstein also provide a model for collaboration that all trainees should consider. Their model was symmetric, basic-clinical scientist collaboration, and a potent model for success in an era of increasing specialization (see commandment 3).

The Nature of Clinical Research

Clinical research is in some cases a unique area of enquiry, and in others, a stepchild of basic research. Clinical research by nature involves the study of patients, either as individual manifestations of disease (case reports) or as populations suffering similar diseases or undergoing treatments (clinical reviews, clinical trials).

At its higher levels, clinical research can gain much recognition and grant income for the institution that is likely to increase as government funding for education decreases and clinical revenue plateaus. A potent example is the Pediatric Oncology Group, now merged as the Clinical Oncology Group. Thanks to collaboration among basic researchers and clinicians at multiple institutions, and the formulation of group protocols (well-defined clinical trials), the five-year-cure rate for childhood acute lymphocytic leukemia has gone from 4% to 60% and is projected to rise to 90% (Medical News Today, 2006). Here is a model for clinical research that can be followed in other subspecialties, first acquiring fellowship training in the diseases and laboratory techniques, then using the opportunity of academic appointment to join appropriate protocols.

Academic primary care physicians and private practitioners can also participate in such collaborations. Programs like those of the American Academy of Pediatrics that fund projects in offices can provide valuable stimulation for practitioners and bring their considerable expertise into the domain of clinical research. Research training during fellowship enhances the physician's ability to interpret clinical research and participate in the academic community. Frances Kelsey was a general practitioner in Canada prior to her administrative position with the FDA, hardly a person expected to advance medical knowledge. Thanks to her appreciation of clinical scholarship and analysis, thousands of children were spared from birth defects because the drug Kevadol (thalidomide) was never approved in the U.S. (Mekdeci, 2011).

NIH Structure and Scientific Review

The primary NIH mission is "to seek fundamental knowledge about the nature and behavior of living systems and the application of that knowledge to enhance health, lengthen life, and reduce the burdens of illness and disability" (Collins, 2010a). An excellent and contemporary description of NIH can be found in Dr. Francis Collins' testimony before Congress shortly after assuming the title of NIH Director (Collins, 2010b). He stated that the institution began as a one-room laboratory in 1887, and now comprises 27 Institutes and Centers, with 80% of its budget devoted to extramural grants supporting research at over 3,000 institutions—including those in 90 countries outside the U.S. NIH employs a two-tiered review process. The first tier is external peer-review panels (study sections), and the second tier is internal advisory councils that fund applications according to study section priority score and their fit with Institute priorities. It is a rigorous, competitive review system that funds approximately one in five grant submissions. The current ~$24 billion annual extramural NIH budget supports 351,000 jobs, with seven high-tech personnel supported in part or in full on the average grant.

Grant application to NIH is now greatly streamlined by electronic communication (NIH, 2009; NIH, 2011a; NIH, 2011b; NIH DPCPSI, 2011, U.S. Department of Health and Human Services, 2011). Invitations to submit applications (NIH, 2011a) are issued based on Institute priorities as parent announcements (PAs) that may include funding opportunity announcements (FOAs) and requests for applications (RFAs). A helpful glossary of NIH terms and abbreviations is provided at their website (NIH, 2011b). There are also NIH-wide initiatives with "trans-NIH research" that includes collaborations on subjects ranging from asthma to autism. These are worth reviewing to note areas of research emphasis and avenues to join in collaborations (NIH DPCPSI, 2011). Lists of active FOAs (NIH, 2011a) and types of NIH grants (U.S. Department of Health and Human Services, 2011) can be reviewed online, allowing selection of the appropriate grant mechanism, registration of the investigator/institution, and submission of a grant proposal. Here is where local agencies designed to promote research, the local Institutional Review Board (IRB), and colleagues experienced with grant submission can be extremely helpful (see Commandments 3 and 7). The most common and prestigious type of grant is the RO1, but young investigator awards and small business grants are worth evaluating for young faculty (U.S. Department of Health and Human Services, 2011).

Those interested in NIH grant support should never decline an opportunity to review grants, whether as part of a regular study section, a specially convened review panel, or as a special consultant. Nothing gives insight into the NIH application and review process like NIH-review participation, and participation in local IRB or research promotion activities is also valuable.

Although NIH is eponymic of federally supported research, it is important to be aware of other sources, like the Department of Defense. Many other agencies fund projects of obvious medical relevance, like research into the toxins and organisms of potential bioterrorism. NIH itself has two main divisions of intramural and extramural research, the former a strong influence (in some opinions a conflicting influence) on research priorities, constitution of review committees, and the review process. The specialized NIH divisions, like pediatrics (NICHD) or heart-lung (NHLI), each have intramural and extramural components, and the administrators developing PAs or review panel appointments often consult their internal scientists. There is thus potential for competition among intramural researchers and extramural grant applications, and it behooves any potential investigator to make as many contacts as possible with intramural NIH researchers and administrators.

The release of a PA from an Institute also initiates a process of review by indicated study sections or Scientific Review Groups (SRG) that will consider the applications. Often these are ongoing groups, like the Mental Retardation Review Committee (under the National Institute of Child Health and Human Development). Occasionally, specialized review committees will be constituted anew or under the aegis of existing study sections, often using special consultants that provide opportunities for review participation. The NIH program administrator invites the committee members and designates one or two as chairs, depending on committee size. Study section members are usually past grantees or those with specialized knowledge about the PA subject, but younger faculty may be selected because of senior faculty obligations, notoriety, and feeling they have already "served their time."

Once applications are received, all go to the Center for Scientific Review at NIH, where 70% (nearly 80,000 applications per year) will be reviewed, using over 17,000 external experts (NIH, 2010; Collins, 2010; NIH, 2011b). The other 30% of applications go to review committees in particular Institutes. An intramural administrator (the Scientific Review Officer or SRO) checks applications for compliance and completeness, recruits members of the Scientific Review Group (SRG), and designates one member as Chair. The SRO coordinates the SRG meetings and the printing/distribution of review critiques. These critiques or summary statements are sent to applicants. They were formerly copied on pink paper and known as pink sheets. The SRO also tries to avoid or mediate conflicts of interest. The SRG chair, usually a distinguished and experienced researcher, moderates the review meeting. The SRO is in attendance to discuss compliance with regulations and administrative issues. The SRO traditionally does not voice opinions on the research. SRG terms are between two to five years, with two to three grant review meetings per year. The confidential applications are sent to SRG members about six weeks before each meeting.

The NIH has expended great effort over the past few years to streamline (enhance) the review process to make it more timely, uniform, and fair. Assessment criteria have been formalized (NIH, 2009; U.S. Department of Health and Human Services, 2011). They include significance, quality of the investigators, innovation, approach, and research environment. Each grant is assigned to a primary and secondary SRG reviewer, and each prepares a critique using forms with the standard headings (U.S. Department of Health and Human Services, 2011). SRG members are typically assigned primary or secondary review for four to six grants per SRG meeting. Additional criteria concerning progress and fulfillment of specific research aims are used for renewal applications, while revised or resubmitted applications are examined for response to prior review critiques. Compliance with NIH extramural research requirements are also evaluated, ranging from human subject or animal protections, inclusion of women/children/minorities, biohazards, and appropriateness of the budget (NIH, 2009; U.S. Department of Health and Human Services, 2011). These requirements are screened by the SRO administrator and examined during the SRG meeting, emphasizing the importance of using local reviewers to scrutinize applications before grant submission. Applicants should have their drafts ready for local review at least two months before grant submission deadlines.

The usual SRG meeting lasts for one to two days. Members present their assigned applications, each beginning with the synopsis and ending with the SRG member's critique. The members read their applications and prepare reviews in a specified format that includes synopsis, critique, and comments on appropriateness of budget, etc. The committee assembles and goes through the applications with the chair(s) as moderator; the two principle reviewers summarize their critiques before the group and recommend approval or disapproval. If approved, a priority score from one (outstanding) to five (unacceptable) is assigned by the principal reviewers. The chair then passes a scoring sheet around, and all members score the grant. The final scoring average, e.g., 1.5, will decide the order of the grant application when it goes to the executive committee. Typically, grants are approved for funding in ascending order on the list until the funds designated for that PA are exhausted. Unfunded applications that are considered adequate are approved and encouraged to re-apply. It is not uncommon for applications to inch up the ladder in subsequent application cycles (decreasing their scores) by addressing reviewer concerns, and ultimately being funded. Those not close to meeting funding criteria are disapproved. Simplifications in the NIH review process are underway to add "not recommended for resubmission" as a signal that the committee had grave reservations about the application (Kaiser, 2008).

The preliminary thought concerning the targeting of your proposal is key to success. Appropriate selection of grant type and NIH institute target requires knowing the expertise and interests of the NIH administrators and "slant" of the institute/section initiating the RFA. This is similar to finding the slant of a medical journal or magazine when you are considering an article submission—the most common complaint of editors is that prospective authors have not read their publication and fail to recognize the journal's scope and preferences. Familiarity with the Institute/administrator/review committee is best done through interaction with colleagues who have submitted grants or served as reviewers with that group. If you have access to individuals in these categories, ask them to read and critique your application, and use institutional research agencies as urged in commandments three and seven.

I will finish this section by pointing to commandment ten: Don't despair. I went through two years and four review cycles before landing an RO1. Although the NIH process of peer review is much superior to earmarks that increasingly intrude into the granting process, there also are weaknesses. Many successful grantees and eventual study section members are basic scientists with no clinical training, and little or no patient experience. PhD psychologists, pharmacologists, and geneticists have many clinical interactions, while a PhD biochemist teaching medical students may have no experience with the clinical arena. Another system weakness is the power of the study section chair in influencing opinion while moderating the reviews. The SRG members who do not review the particular grant are heavily dependent on the comments of the principal reviewers and the study section head. A final weakness is the difficulty in attracting knowledgeable reviewers to travel to two to three study section meetings per year. Chairs are sometimes forced to rely on young scientists with little review experience.

Another concern is my opinion that clinical scholarship is not recognized as valid clinical research that can be considered for federal funding. Patients are the elements of clinical medicine, encounters that teach us the relations of history, physical, and differential diagnosis, and infuse the contexts of clinic, hospital ward, and medical home. Therefore, case presentations are the essence of clinical medicine. Grand rounds or case conferences showing case presentations are models of medical insight in the way that scientific advances are Homeric for basic research.

Every disease begins as a case report, its spectrum and optimal management defined by more case reports. The case report is to clinical trial as the pure culture is to mixed flora, each having value.

It is important for medical school administrators and promotion committees to recognize case reports as the equivalent of basic or clinical research, all advancing knowledge.

Ten Commandments for Grant Success

1. Know yourself. Just as it is important to select your medical specialty and your preference for teaching or practice, it is important to assess your talents and preparation for research. If you sought time in the laboratory in college, medical school, and residency/fellowship, then you have potential for the basic research that absorbs most of the NIH budget. Important here is whether you had the autonomy to pursue your own directions and experiments, for those physicians who are destined to be good investigators (rather than good technicians) will have demanded input into their work. If you are more interested in evidence-based medicine and clinical trials, with a talent for precise analysis and statistics, then clinical research will be opportune. Realize that applying a few laboratory techniques to a particular disease or collating cases can satisfy clinical scholarship, but never the standards of NIH review.

2. Protect your time. Young faculty at medical schools are often besieged by requests, such as lectures, course directorships, committees, and hospital positions, which all seem prestigious until recognized as off-loading by senior faculty. View early faculty years as a residency in grant application and laboratory establishment. If federal funding is your aim, then respectfully decline all time-consuming opportunities not necessary for your practice. The demands of clinical knowledge and practice added to research expertise makes it difficult for physicians to compete, and it is easy to underuse your start-up funds when duties limit your lab time to a weekly technician meeting. Negotiation with your chair and division director should have allocated time for research, a task made easier if you have fulfilled commandment 1 with publications appropriate to your goals. Never accept an appointment in a division with fewer than three members, and ensure that a reasonable clinical load will be accommodated for at least three to four years.

3. Reach out. This seems to be in conflict with commandment 2, but academic isolation is death to faculty growth. Choose obligations that promote the flow of grant information and scientific interaction. A lecture in the medical biochemistry course may be valuable if it brings contact with seasoned grantees and potential collaborators; scheduling grand rounds may be worthwhile if you partner with fabled Dr. X whose grants are legion. Always attend your departmental research conferences and make your presence and interests known. Although your research may overshadow projects of less current faculty, avoid arrogance, and share their knowledge of local and NIH systems. Most importantly, make contact with other research faculty and learn about available equipment and core facilities. Most physicians achieve only a few years of grant funding, after which these collaborations can generate satisfying clinical scholarship.

4. Think broadly, write narrowly. One of the most difficult tasks faced by young faculty is the trimming of their voluminous ideas into succinct, stepwise inquiries. Most successful grants will have succinct hypotheses with yes or no answers, including preliminary results that outline a logical path to those answers.

5. If you aim high, avoid crossroads. A young investigator with established instruments or laboratory techniques will often encounter serendipitous opportunities, either as opportune collaborations (your lung tissue with her membrane protein assay) or clinic visits (your hepatitis patients with his bile acid measures). Sometimes these can be profitable and career-changing; more likely they will submerge your major project below funding levels. On the other hand, selective collaborations or case studies can build your CV towards promotion and secure relationships that place you as co-investigator on others' grants. Synthetic thinking is necessary and natural for clinicians, so pursuing diverse opportunities may reveal that you are more suited for clinical scholarship and research collaboration than for headline NIH research. Seize the citations and recognize yourself.

6. Know NIH. There has been a vast improvement in the transparency of NIH workings thanks to the Internet and NIH administrators. The NIH mission, structure, research priorities, review criteria, and grant submission instructions/forms are all available on the web (NIH, 2009; NIH, 2011a; NIH, 2010, Collins, 2010, NIH, 2011b; U.S. Department of Health and Human Services, 2011). Invitations for investigator-initiated research are listed (NIH, 2010), along with "trans-NIH" collaborations, indicating priority areas (NIH, 2011b) and the types of grants available (NIH, 2011a). The procedures of SRGs or study sections are now formalized with specific review criteria and formats (NIH, 2009; U.S. Department of Health and Human Services, 2011), and there is even a sample SRG meeting available on You-Tube (NIH, 2009). Translating this information into action for grant proposals will be greatly aided by local experts, re-emphasizing the dictum of Commandment 3.

7. Prepare well, write early, and revise often. As mentioned in commandment nine, review PAs, and whenever possible, discuss them with NIH administrators. Approach administrators at meetings or even with cold calls, as most will encourage young faculty toward investigation. Look for subtle language in the PA that may indicate preference for types of investigators (like neuroscientists) or specific approaches (like stem cells). Procrastination affects most of us, particularly busy clinician scholars or investigators, so subtract six months from any grant deadline. The assembly of preliminary results and the early framing of the hypotheses, specific aims, and objectives are essential for a logical, focused, and feasible proposal. Most institutions have research staff that can help with Institutional Review Board and NIH requirements, and many have experienced science writers who can optimize proposals when received in time.

8. Don't get angry, get educated. If you aspire to NIH funding, use any means to participate in NIH review, whether as the lowest one-time technical expert or a regular study section member with its considerable time commitment. This demonstrates your commitment, and gives you invaluable

information on the review process (not to mention first-name basis with NIH administrators). Call or get to know your program administrator before submission and call them afterwards to clarify critiques or assess the mood of the review, but never protest angrily. They work very hard and have many to satisfy.

9. Write and rewrite. Most new proposals will not be funded at first review, almost as a rite of passage by veterans reluctant to laud a rookie. In the spirit of Commandment 8, read your critique carefully. If your grant was approved, but not funded, follow the recommendations precisely: A major part of resubmission review is to assess how well the investigator responded to criticisms. Most revisions will gradually decrease the priority score and allow the grant to be funded. If your grant was disapproved, then rethink your approach. Consult with your local experts and consider if your training and your time commitment allow research that will outshine 80% of your peers, even more since clinical grants have historically had lower funding rates (Brinkley, 1999).

10. Don't despair. If you have received rejections and feel you have the talent and leadership to run projects at the NIH level, then keep writing. Other federal agencies and local charities can sustain a laboratory, and there are many scientific discoveries made later in life. However, there is life after NIH grant failure, for your research experience gives you informed knowledge of your specialty literature and many opportunities for clinical collaboration and scholarship. You will have to decide how long to strive for NIH funding, dictated in part by Commandments one and two.

13 | Industry and Philanthropy

Michael E. Okogbo, MD, MBA

The funding process begins with identifying funding sources that match your research question (Thomson, 2007). The nature and design of your research project and the assessment and search for funding are intimately linked (Mackway-Jones, 2003). An accurate assessment of funding will require a good grasp of the research to be undertaken and a proper understanding of the necessary time course of the project.

Once the research project has been designed, the next question to answer is whether there is a need for funding. Some research projects may not need external funding, while others may require a huge financial outlay. Answer the following questions (Mackway-Jones, 2003):

1. Will extra staff time be necessary for this work?
2. Will extra equipment be needed?
3. Will extra consumables be needed?

4. Is funding in place for your literature review and secretarial time?

5. Will there be charges for statistical and health economic support?

6. Will other departments need to provide resources for this work?

If any of the answers are yes, then funding will be needed; the degree will depend on the number of affirmatives. Categories in estimating costs are: staff, equipment, consumables, research support, administrative support, and miscellaneous.

Staff: The questions to address are the number of hours per week required to complete the work required and the expertise of the person required to do the work. The professional background of the researcher will affect the bill. In general, researchers with a medical background cost more than those with other training. The individuals to be supported by the funding must have the professional background and experience to operate at the level required for the research project.

Equipment: Funders look closely at requests for equipment funding. It is essential to think through this request carefully.

Consumables: Try to identify all consumables. The best way to capture these is to imagine the path of a particular patient through the research process. Each item that is used in the pathway can then be identified and the cost estimated.

Research support: This includes statistical services, specialist input like health economics or computer modeling. If the researcher's institution has research support for certain aspects of the project, then a request for outside funding may not be necessary.

Administrative Support & Miscellany: Every research project will need some administrative support, including secretarial staff, office space, and accounts management. A realistic assessment for these needs has to be made to decide if existing resources can handle the administrative load. Similarly, miscellany can often be overlooked. These expenses include job advertisements, travel to meetings, stipends for subjects, and conference fees.

If outside funding is necessary, the next task is to find a funding body willing to foot the bill. A good rule of thumb is to get advice from researchers already active in your area of interest (Mackway-Jones, 2003). Is collaboration with a more experienced researcher an option? An advantage of this is that it enhances the chances of success if young investigators team up with established researchers. Excellent Internet resources are now available, e.g., http://www.rdinfo.org.uk/, http://foundationcenter.org.

Funding Environment

There are three major sources of funding for biomedical research: the government, private (philanthropic) foundations, and industry.

The NIH is the major source of government funding for research, but there are other government agencies that fund research. The Centers for Disease Control and Prevention, the United States Department of Agriculture, the National Science Foundation, the Veterans Administration, the Department of Defense, and the National Aeronautics and Space Administration are some other government agencies that support research (Anonymous, 2007).

Current trends indicate that there is a general stabilization of government funding for research and an increasing reliance on foundations and industry for research dollars (Anonymous, 2007; Wadman, 2007). Private, non-corporate support for biomedical research in the U.S. grew by 36%, from $1.8 billion to $2.5 billion between 1994 and 2003 (Moses, Dorsey, Matheson, & Thier, 2005). There are indications that this trend is still on the upswing.

Be that as it may, philanthropic funding for research is not more than 5% of the $100 billion spent on biomedical research in the U.S. annually. The biotechnology and pharmaceutical industries account for 60% of the money spent on biomedical research (Wadman, 2007). The philanthropists or gigaphilanthropists, as some writers now refer to them, fill the gaps left by government and industry. According to science writer Meredith Wadman, "They dictate exactly what their money should be spent on, and act quickly compared with the sometimes glacial pace of government agencies" (Wadman, 2007). This is because they have flexibility with spending that industry and government agencies do not have. They are not answerable to shareholders or venture capitalists, nor do they labor under the political scrutiny experienced by NIH and other government agencies.

The Bill and Melinda Gates Foundation, Howard Hughes Medical Institute, and the Wellcome Trust of the UK are major players in this league. The Bill and Melinda Gates Foundation, considered the largest grant-making foundation in the world (Renz & Atienza, 2006), has three main programs: a U.S. program that focuses on secondary and post-secondary education, a global development program that focuses on hunger and poverty, and a global health program. Of the $2.1 billion that the Foundation provided for its programs in 2007, $1.2 billion (61%) went to global health initiatives (Bill and Melinda Gates Foundation, 2007). The Wellcome Trust is an unsung hero in health research and comes second to the Bill and Melinda Gates Foundation in the amount it spends on biomedical research. In 2008, the Trust announced increased spending on biomedical research to four billion pounds over the next five years, an increase of 60% (*Lancet* Editorial, 2008). Most of the Trust's funds are used in the UK, but it also supports research efforts in resource-poor countries of Asia and Africa. The Trust is engaged in two global partnerships, the SNP consortium, a not-for-profit organization based in the U.S., and the International HapMap Project, involving scientists and funding agencies from Canada, China, Japan, Nigeria, and the U.S. Both global partnerships are involved in genome research into single nucleotide polymorphisms (SNPs) and combinations of SNPs that are inherited together (haplotypes).

The role of foundations in biomedical research has come under criticism lately because of the huge amount of money that they use to support non-governmental organizations, policy tanks, and universities. Some worry that it confers a tremendous amount of clout on the foundations and, therefore, significant leverage in policy-making and agenda-setting in civil society, nationally, and globally (McCoy, Kembhavi, Patel, & Luintel, 2009).

However, there are those who think these philanthropies are not doing enough–that they should provide leadership, vision, and resources to ensure the wealth of knowledge available about health is used to develop policies, practices and programs that will improve the future health of the population (Gruman & Prager, 2002). Thus, rather than allocating grants for development of new technologies, they should be supporting research on how to overcome barriers to use of existing technologies (Leroy, 2006). In this regard, some suggest that they should focus on public health needs, develop and support trans-disciplinary research, contribute to increased flexibility in the research environment, and work to broaden the focus of federal research funding. As a strategic agenda, philanthropy should help both the government and academic health sciences to more closely connect their investments in research with their payoff in improved health (Gruman & Prager, 2002).

Eligibility

When looking for an appropriate funding opportunity, investigate the eligibility requirements of the grant. The granting body usually states what the eligibility criteria are. Criteria would include academic and practice status of the applicant, e.g., MD, DO, PhD. The nationality of the applicant or immigration status of the applicant may also be a criterion. The research grant may be for young investigators or those at a certain career stage.

Funding Sources

The government remains a major source of funding for research. However, the gap that the government does not cover is filled by industry and philanthropy. Industry essentially means biotechnology and pharmaceutical companies, which are important sources for research dollars. There are always ethical issues to consider when getting research grants from industry because industry partners may have a biased interest in the outcome of the research.

Although foundations and not-for-profit organizations are good sources for research dollars, there are risks associated with this source. There is the possibility of discontinuation of funding at short notice, and proprietary property may or may not belong to the researcher or his institution (Thomson, 2007). Some funders demand a level of accountability that can make some researchers uncomfortable; funders do not write a check and walk away to leave the researcher on his own (Wadman, 2007). For a list of philanthropic funding sources, see

Foundation Center (2011) and the Council on Foundations (COS, 2011). These bodies collate and share data regarding grant support for over 2,000 organizations. The information they provide includes the interests of the organization, funding amounts, grant application processes and forms, lists of peer–reviewed publications resulting from previously funded research, as well as contact information for each organization. A limited search of their data can be conducted free of charge, but for a more comprehensive search, a fee is required.

Funding Opportunities: Staying Informed and Tips for Funding Success

There are several search engines and web sites to access to stay informed on grant opportunities; www.grants.gov is a good place to start. Other places to look include Community of Science Funding Opportunities (COS, 2011), Research Research (Research, 2011), and U.S. Department of Health and Human Services Grants Net (2011b).

Other methods of staying informed include attending scientific meetings, participation in research-related list-serves, and professional collaborations and networking. Keep in touch with your institution's research office, if it has one.

Tips for success in research grant funding: (Thomson, 2007)

- Find the right foundation that matches your needs - this is imperative.

- Submit a well-designed letter to the funding source, with a proposal that is consistent with the organization's funding goals.

- Allow sufficient time for preparation and local review before submission (12 months is optimal).

- Identify an appropriate mentor and describe the mentoring plan for the grant submission process.

- Follow guidelines closely in writing the proposal, as most funding organizations tend to be fastidious about this.

- Be explicit as to the significance of the research in advancing science, clinical practice, or public health.

- Avoid an overly ambitious proposal, instead stay focused.

- Meet deadlines. Most organizations reject proposals submitted after stated deadlines.

- Read the reviewer guidelines to understand the criteria that will be applied in reviewing each application.

- Review any published/database of current and previously funded research.

- Contact the granting agency research administrator to discuss your proposal in advance to gain insight on relevance to the funding source's priorities.

- Be persistent. If rejected for funding, be responsive to the reviewer critiques and resubmit in a timely manner.

Remember that funding bodies are asking themselves two questions: (Mackway, 2003)

1. Is the research question worth answering?

2. Can the applicant successfully answer the question?

As a final check, read through the proposal and ask these questions yourself. If the answer to either is no, then start again.

14 | Scientific Presentations

E.F. Luckstead, MD
Roger D. Smalligan, MD, MPH

Scientific data can be presented in the form of an abstract, poster presentation, oral presentation, or a written manuscript. Scientific writing for publication will be described in a subsequent chapter. Scientific meetings provide opportunities for investigators to present case reports and original research to their peers. The meetings are also excellent opportunities to exchange ideas with like-minded colleagues and to form alliances that can influence career paths.

Isolated case reports often represent a student's first presentation and subsequent publication. Increasingly sophisticated presentations are expected at the resident, fellow, and faculty levels. Local, regional, and national/international meetings warrant increasingly higher expectations for scientific presentation.

In all instances, concise but descriptive presentations are the goal. Verbosity should be avoided and adept use of tables and figures is essential. Seeking out a faculty mentor who has experience in scientific writing and presentation is invaluable and greatly increases the chances of success in the entire process (Ogunyemi, Solnik,

Alexander, Fong, & Azziz, 2010). This is especially important if the presenter speaks English as a second language (Cameron, Chang & Pagel, 2011).

Abstracts – The Entry Point

Scientific meetings of each of the different medical specialties and subspecialties typically have a "Call for Abstracts," which is announced several months prior to the meeting. Many societies have meetings on both a regional and national level. There are also opportunities at a local and state level in certain specialties or universities. Some meetings invite only research abstracts, which means they are interested in descriptions of new or ongoing research projects that may provide preliminary or final data from a study. Other meetings also welcome case report or "clinical vignette" abstracts. This latter category is the most common entry point for students, residents, and junior faculty to begin presenting at scientific meetings. The likelihood of having an abstract accepted varies greatly, depending most of all on the quality of the abstract, but also on a particular meeting's scope of interest, notoriety, and number of submissions. The larger, more well-known meetings are the most difficult to gain acceptance. Regional meetings will often accept the majority of well-written abstract submissions because the goal of the organizers is to increase participation of the membership and to allow a venue for junior investigators to gain experience. Larger national meetings may have an intense review process that selects only the most unique cases or research projects. Many regional meetings and most national meetings will typically publish accepted abstracts as a supplement to their journal, which is a nice bonus for the researcher, as this can be listed on one's curriculum vitae as a "Published Abstract."

Depending on the meeting's format, the highest rated abstracts will be chosen for "Oral Presentation," with the next level of accepted submissions being deemed appropriate for a "Poster Presentation." Some meetings or sessions are restricted to "Poster Presentation" only, and some investigators prefer the poster format because it fosters free communication and exchange of ideas among authors and interested researchers.

The Clinical Vignette or Case Report Abstract

The clinical vignette abstract is easy to write after identifying an appropriate case to write about. The key is to find a case that is unique, extremely rare, or an unusual variation of a more common condition. You want a topic that will pique the interest of your audience. The end-product will be a 350-700 word abstract that begins with a section describing the case and is followed by a discussion or teaching section. The exact length and format are described in the meeting's "Call for Abstracts." The case description should be very similar to what would be presented during busy work rounds at the hospital: a brief history of the present illness that includes an appropriate review of systems points, past medical history, physical exam, laboratory and x-ray findings, diagnosis, and hospital course. The discussion section begins with a brief description of the condition, its usual epidemiology, usual presentation, available therapy, and usual outcomes. Specific references to the case and how it fits the profile or deviates from usual norms should be highlighted. Write clearly, eliminate typos, use accepted grammar, and avoid unusual abbreviations (Hines, Wible, & McCartney, 2010). The final touch is a catchy title. The best title is often a play on words that encapsulates the most interesting aspect of the case (Byrne, 1998). For example, a complicated patient with polyneuropathy who was ultimately determined to have POEMS syndrome might be entitled "A POEM Without Rhyme or Reason." The following is a sample clinical vignette abstract that was accepted for presentation at a recent regional meeting:

A Real Pain – The Danger of Discitis

Case Report: A 53-year-old man with a history of nephrolithiasis presented with several days of sharp pain in the right flank. Pain was worse with movement and better if laying on his left side. He had subjective fevers but no chills and denied hematuria, dysuria, or frequency. PE: T 100.7° F; right flank pain and RLQ abdominal tenderness, and obturator sign was positive. Lab: WBC 13.3 x 10³; neutrophils 87.5%; Hgb 14.7; UA positive for blood and bacteria. Abdominal CT showed no stones, obstruction, or appendicitis. Antibiotics were started immediately, but fever persisted for two days.

Re-examination showed point tenderness in the lumbar spine. Blood cultures grew MRSA. ESR was 58 and CRP was 112. MRI showed inflammation and disk herniation at L5-S1 confirming discitis. Neurosurgery was consulted and performed a laminectomy with debridement. The patient had a slow but full recovery.

Discussion: Back pain is one of the most common presenting complaints in the clinic and emergency department. A readily identifiable benign cause is found in the vast majority of cases. Our patient's initial evaluation required multiple diagnoses to be ruled out including nephrolithiasis, pyelonephritis, septic arthritis, and appendicitis. The spinal tenderness and persistent fever led to the correct diagnosis of discitis. Discitis occurs in approximately one in 450,000 patients and is closely associated with vertebral osteomyelitis. The incidence increases with age, and is more common in men than women. The most frequent cause is hematogenous spread of infection to bone which erodes into the disc space. Other routes include contiguous spread from infected tissue or trauma, including surgery or instrumentation. This case is unusual as the pain was acute; usually it begins insidiously and worsens over weeks to months. The mean duration of symptoms is 48 days before diagnosis. MRI is the most sensitive study for detection. Staphylococcus aureus is the cause in more than 50% of cases, with Streptococci and Gram negative rods following. Treatment with IV antibiotics alone is sometimes sufficient; however, surgery is necessary in complicated cases. Although mortality is only 5% in the modern era, early recognition is critical to prevent long term neurologic sequelae.

Research Abstracts

Writing a research abstract demands efficiency of prose and effective communication. The research abstract always begins with a short description of the "Purpose of the Study" or important

"Background Information" to set the stage for the study and describe its relevance. Next is the "Methods" section, where exactly what was done and what information was gathered is detailed. Statistical methods are included. The following section is entitled "Results" and presents the findings (often in tabular form). The final section of the research abstract is entitled "Conclusions," where the meaning and significance of the results are summarized. The title of a research abstract should be as descriptive as possible. The following is an example of a research abstract:

CONTROL ID: 747453

PRESENTATION TYPE: Oral Presentation

CATEGORY: Health Care Research

TITLE: ADHERENCE TO DEMENTIA GUIDELINES IN THE TEXAS PANHANDLE

AUTHORS (FIRST NAME, LAST NAME): Mohammed Samiuddin[1], Maria Teresa Ranin[2], Stephanie C McClure[2], Roger D Smalligan[2]

INSTITUTIONS (ALL): 1. Family Medicine, Texas Tech University Health Sciences Center, Amarillo, TX, USA.
2. Internal Medicine, Texas Tech Health Sciences Center, Amarillo, TX, USA.

ABSTRACT BODY:
Purpose of Study: Dementia is the leading cause of disability among older adults. Alzheimer's disease (AD) comprises 55% to 77% of all dementia diagnoses. Studies show that dementia is the most significant risk factor for institutionalization and currently more than 1.5 million Americans reside in nursing homes. This number is expected to more than triple by the year 2030. The Alzheimer's Association developed the Best Practices of Dementia Care Guidelines in 2006 for nursing homes, and they have been adopted by the U.S. Department of Health and Human Services. This study was designed to assess the adherence rate of Texas Panhandle nursing homes to these current guidelines and to identify opportunities for improvement.

Methods Used: Surveys were sent to all 34 nursing homes in the Texas Panhandle that were officially listed. The online survey had 44 questions presented in a multiple-choice format and were analyzed using Microsoft Excel.

Summary of Results: 20 of 34 (59%) nursing homes had administrators or MDS Coordinators complete the survey. Nursing homes reported an average of 45 (range 2-100) residents with the diagnosis of dementia. Responses to key questions about "Best Practices of Dementia Care" included: 1) screening for dementia and depression upon admission to the facility: 50% (goal 100% for all); 2) of those that do screen, only 32% repeat screening after a significant behavior change is noted; 3) close monitoring of residents on some type of mood stabilizing agent or antipsychotic medication: 45%; 4) training of staff about falls and pressure ulcers: 100%; 5) advance care planning: 100%; 6) recreational activities for residents: 100%; 7) knowledge of local support groups for families: 41%; 8) willing to have staff attend in-service training every 1-3 months: 72%.

Conclusions: This study suggests that while certain aspects of the "Best Practices" are being employed by area nursing homes, there remain some important deficiencies. Fortunately, the survey shows great openness on the part of the majority of nursing homes towards learning more about the guidelines and improving care for this growing population of residents with dementia. Educational activities should be provided as soon as is feasible for these interested facilities.

Oral Presentations

The most highly ranked abstracts will be selected for oral presentation. These may be clinical vignettes or research abstracts, depending on the meeting and category chosen. Oral presentations should reflect the core points of the presentation with an introduction, an outline listing three or four major concepts, slides with pertinent tables or figures that are easily readable, and a summary or concluding "take-home" message. Prepare for the talk by producing a series of electronic slides that will serve as prompts for the oral presentation. Slides with bullet points of the key topics jog the memory of the presenter and keep the presentation on pace. Ideally, no more than four or five bullet points per slide, with a running title at the top for a given section, helps keep the listener oriented. Avoid complete sentences (Browner, 1999). Include as many graphics (diagrams, photos, x-rays, graphs) as appropriate to make your point. Explain each verbally and keep them simple. The order of the presentation and the abstract are similar, but additional information can be added to the talk. Abide by the time limit and allow time for questions at the end. A good rule of thumb is one slide per minute. References and acknowledgements of those who assisted in the work should be given on the final slides. It is always a good idea to practice your oral presentation with an audience who will provide constructive criticism.

At many meetings, the audience will be small and consist mainly of presenters. Hence, it is often a warm and interested audience. Relax and talk to the audience rather than stare at the slides. Keep the pace quick, but not rushed. Speak clearly and distinctly. Try to avoid verbal fillers, such as "um" and "you know" (Shelledy, 2004). Do not pace or stand frozen at the lectern, and use humor if appropriate (Hemphill, 2009). At the break, try to speak with faculty or residents who have shown an interest in your topic. Show respect to your colleagues as they present and ask cogent questions. This can be an excellent opportunity to make contacts and network.

Poster Presentations

Poster presentations are an important part of almost every meeting. This is also an honor and requires significant preparation to produce a good product. Poster presentations are expanded abstracts, with succinct descriptions and summaries, and illustrated with helpful graphics. Always apply the *KISS principle* – keep it simple and informative.

The goal is to communicate your research or case review findings clearly and succinctly to an audience who will probably only spend a few minutes in front of your poster (Depoy & Gitlin, 1998). Most meetings provide specific instructions about the size of the poster and any specific information that should be included. A standard poster is approximately four feet by six feet and fits nicely on the standard presentation board that the society will provide for you to mount your poster on the day of the meeting (the presentation board stands on legs and is usually four feet by eight feet).

The organization of the poster is the same as the abstract (Shelledy, 2004). Some meetings prefer that the poster begin with "Learning Objectives," while others start with the **History and Physical** for a vignette or with the **Background** for a research project. The abstract itself should not be included on the poster unless specifically requested in the instructions. Keep complete sentences to a minimum on a poster. Bullet points that present the essential information succinctly are the key to a good poster, along with attractive photos and graphics. Always seek the advice of others and proof-read the poster several times to avoid embarrassing mistakes. Be sure that the text is easy to read and that several photos or illustrations are used to make the poster as visually appealing as possible. Use a font size that is easily readable from a few feet from the poster, typically at least size 36, but somewhat larger is also good. In general, use the same font and size in all of the text sections of your poster. Three to five references cited in the background or discussion and presented in the accepted format should be included at the end of the poster. The font size of this section can be considerably smaller to save space.

If your institution offers professional graphic arts services, you are in luck. Provide the text in a word processing document, along with files containing the pertinent photos and graphics to be included. The designer will return a draft for review and corrections before final printing. If no professional assistance is available, prepare the poster as a single slide in Microsoft PowerPoint® by cutting and pasting the appropriate materials and text. The slide can be printed at a commercial printing/copy company or can be sent to a commercial poster printing site on-line. Glossy paper is good, but lamination causes problems in handling and mounting.

On the day of the presentation, arrive at the designated time to mount the poster. Bring push pins in case the meeting does not supply them. Dress professionally and stand proudly by your poster during the hours designated by the meeting. Greet passers-by and offer to give a brief explanation of the key points of your poster if they show interest. Limit your oral presentation to two to four minutes unless there are questions. Some meetings will have designated judges approach each poster to rate it, and many meetings provide a prize for the best poster(s).

Poster presentations offer a wonderful opportunity for students, residents, and investigators at all levels to meet new people, especially those with common interests. Program directors and chairs often attend these meetings with an eye for potential candidates for their programs. As time allows, be sure to visit other posters at the session to gather ideas for future presentations. For a sample poster, see Figure 14.1.

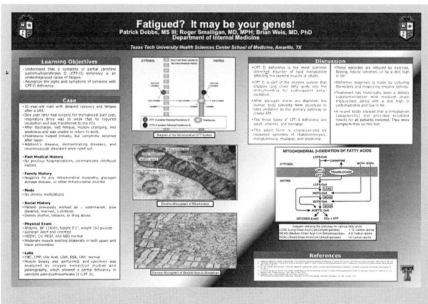

Figure 14.1. Sample of Poster Presentation

15 | Writing for Scientific Publication

Candace A. Myers, PhD

You have completed your project or made an observation, so the next step is to share the information with the medical community. Our scientific method for distributing scholarly work is through publication in peer-reviewed journals. Today's journals are a mix of printed and online articles. A case report is frequently a young author's first foray into publication. Many of the publication considerations for a case report are the same as for an original research article. For this discussion, we will describe the steps involved in submitting an original research article for publication, and then go back and describe the submission of a case report.

The important steps to successful publication in a peer-reviewed medical journal are:

1. Journal selection

2. Composition

3. Proof reading and revision

4. Submission

5. Acceptance

Journal Selection

Identifying a journal is easier if you are a regular reader of the journals in your medical specialty. You will consider the journals that reach your target audience. Consider the journals that have previously published articles on the general topic of your manuscript.

Most reputable journals are peer-reviewed. When an article is submitted to a peer-reviewed journal, it is first evaluated by the editor for relevance, quality, timeliness, and style. If the editor thinks the article is appropriate for his/her journal, the manuscript is sent to reviewers who are experts in the field. The editor selects the appropriate reviewers based on their knowledge of the subject and their willingness to review an article at the time. The reviewers read the submitted manuscript and send their comments and suggestions for improvement to the editor. If after reading the reviewers' comments the editor is still interested in publishing the manuscript, he/she will return it to the author with the reviewers' comments and a request to make changes in line with the reviewers' consensus.

Authors typically aspire to publish their papers in the most prestigious and well-known journals. These journals have high impact factors, which are the average number of recent citations per article published in the journal. Impact factors vary from year-to-year and are only one metric used to rate medical journals.

Composition

Each journal publishes INSTRUCTIONS TO AUTHORS. These instructions are usually available from a journal's home page and describe the specific directions authors should follow when submitting a manuscript for consideration. They include a formatting guide and differ for each journal. Most journals will publish original articles, review articles, case reports, and correspondence. Different instructions and word limits apply for each type of article.

In general, authors should strive for brevity, clarity, accuracy, and completeness. Research reports are reports of past occurrences; therefore, most of each manuscript should be worded in the past tense. The discussion may be submitted in the present tense. In the past, scientific literature was usually written in the passive voice because it was considered to be objective, impersonal, and well-suited to science writing. Today most journals prefer the active voice.

Examples:

Passive Voice: The samples were analyzed by Smith et al.

Active Voice: Smith et al. analyzed the samples.

Most manuscript submissions are made online. The information that traditionally was included in the cover page is now entered into the appropriate boxes during the submission process. You will need a clear descriptive title that contains no abbreviations. Some journals also request a running title, which is a shortened version of the title that can be used in the header on subsequent pages of the article. They will ask for the full names of each author. Authors should use a consistent spelling of their name with their middle initial, so that the author's body of work can be grouped properly on PubMed. You will need the names of the authors' institutions and perhaps the authors' degrees. The journal may ask for the authors' titles and their positions at their institutions. One author will be named as the corresponding author, and he/she must provide contact information. Acknowledgements may be solicited. Here you can list the names of the people who helped with the study, data collection, editing the manuscript, or the statistics. The source of financial support for the work is also listed on the cover page.

You will need to write an abstract that succinctly summarizes the purpose of the study, procedures used, findings, statistical significance, main conclusions, and implications of the conclusions. Abstracts are often limited to 150-250 words. The abstract is a stand-alone summary of the entire project and allows readers to sift through many articles in a relatively short period of time. Although the abstract is placed at the beginning of a scientific article, it should be the last section composed. A list of three to five key words is typically included after the abstract. The keywords cover the main topics discussed in the article and should be selected from the Medical Subject Headings (MESH) in Index Medicus (http://www.nlm.nih.gov/mesh/MBrowser.html).

When writing an original research manuscript, rely on your protocol and the paper will be half written. Your manuscript will usually include:

- Introduction/background
- Hypotheses
- Methods
- Results
- Graphics
- Discussion
- Conclusions
- References

Refer to a recent article in the journal you selected to serve as a guide when writing your submission.

Introduction/Background

The Introduction/Background clearly states the problem or premise with adequate background information to allow an intelligent reader to understand your research report. This section includes a review of pertinent articles leading to the conduct of your study and defines terms used in the manuscript. The goals and objectives of the study and the rationale for conducting the study should be explained. You can begin with the introduction/background from the protocol and update it with literature that has been published since your protocol was written. You will need to state your hypothesis(ses). This is where you go out on a limb and state the premise you set out to prove by conducting the research.

Methods

The methods section should be written with sufficient detail for a skilled investigator to reproduce the study. Begin by describing your study design. Explain how subjects were recruited and what eligibility criteria had to be met. Describe how the subjects were randomized and to what extent the study was blinded. Explain how the blinding was accomplished.

The next portion of the methods section should describe the interventions that were studied. This discussion should include information about doses, controls (placebo or standard of care), and duration of treatment. A schematic that graphically explains the study groups and study activities, and how data were collected over time might be included. Methods include a complete listing of the variables measured and the modes of analysis. If you are duplicating exactly a method cited in another article, reference that article for a description of the method, and save the publisher some space. Equipment and reagents should be mentioned. Manufacturers with their city, state, and country should be included in parentheses. Describe the statistical tests applied to the data and name the relevant level of significance.

Results

Present the research results in a logical order. A summary of the subject's demographics are often presented first to demonstrate the effectiveness of the randomization in producing groups with similar mean characteristics at study initiation. Tables and figures can be inserted to summarize the data. Mention each graphic in the text of the manuscript (Figure 1 or Table 1). If data are presented graphically, there is no need to repeat the same information in the text of the manuscript. Include both negative and unexpected results. The convention is to display control data followed by intervention data. Acknowledge any problems or deviations in the data collection process. Do not include any reference citations or discussion of your findings in the results section. Provide the facts, just the facts.

In the printed article, the graphic components will be interspersed throughout the text, but for online submission, the tables and figures are usually managed as separate files. The captions for the graphics are often in yet another file. The author instructions about graphics are often very specific, but some details can be ironed out after the manuscript is accepted.

Discussion

The discussion is the heart of the article. Describe, in an orderly fashion, what the results mean. Refer to the graphic presentations and point out specific aspects about the population studied. Emphasize new and important findings. Use the discussion to interpret your results in light of what is already known, and describe other relevant studies and how they relate or compare to your results. Did you achieve your goals? Was your hypothesis proven? Discuss all the debatable aspects of your results. What is the next step? Describe your future work. Summarize the strengths and limitations of the study.

Conclusions

Some journals have a conclusion in addition to the discussion. End with a summation of the study conclusions.

References

Claims made in the introduction/background and discussion, and sources of methodology should be referenced with individual reputable literature sources. Most references are other peer-reviewed journal articles, but books and websites may also be cited. When a claim is made or a method is first mentioned in the text of your manuscript, you should insert a citation that directs the reader to the source for the original article. The citation note in the text is usually a superscript number at the end of the sentence where the claim is made. The submission journal's instructions to authors will describe the format used by the journal. Reference management software (RefWorks or EndNotes®) can be very useful in tracking the references during the writing/revision process and is available free at many institutions through site licenses.

Suitable reference materials are found in peer-reviewed journals, books, and websites. Use actual source documents, not review articles that cite original findings. When using Internet resources, remember that Wikipedia is NEVER an acceptable source document and services that require subscriptions and fees are not available to your reader, so they should not be cited.

Publishers will have legal concerns about the materials you provide. Some journals will require a copy of the release from a subject whose images are used in an article. Permission to use copyrighted material is always necessary. Conventions exist to block the faces of subjects to protect their anonymity. Care must be taken to prevent the reuse of other author's phraseology. Computer programs exist to identify plagiarized text.

Proof Reading and Revision

Allow time for sufficient proof reading and revision of your manuscript draft. It is often good to let your manuscript rest for a few days, and then read it with fresh eyes. You will be surprised by the number of details you missed the first time through. When you proof, pay attention to syntax, tenses, punctuation, and spelling. Be consistent. Minimize the use of jargon and eliminate any empty phrases. Use the spell checker and the grammar checker on your word processor. Check all your calculations and note any trademarked or registered products properly. Ask your mentor and trusted colleagues to read your article and offer constructive criticism. Publishers are concerned about space, so eliminate any redundancy and be concise in your use of language.

Submission and Acceptance

Online submission is usually tedious and time-consuming. Allot sufficient time to check all your work before you hit the SUBMIT button. The submission software usually alerts you when your submission is successfully received. The wait to learn the fate of your submission can be weeks to months. The editor could reject it very quickly. If the editor sends it to reviewers, they are often asked to return it in two weeks, but it may take them longer. The editor may have trouble locating reviewers willing and able to review the article, thereby delaying a decision. Few articles are accepted as they are submitted. Most manuscripts that are eventually published are returned to the author with suggestions and comments from the reviewers.

Case Report

A case report is frequently the first article submitted for publication by a medical student or resident. It arises because something surprising occurred in the clinic or hospital. Cases are often found worthy of publication if:

- They are extremely rare occurrences.
- They involve an unexpected adverse response to common therapy.
- They question current therapy.
- They illustrate an unusual combination of events.
- They present a combination of symptoms that confuse the decision-making process.
- They involve a profound experience that results in a reevaluation of a medical treatment.

Stay alert for cases that fit one of these categories. When you recognize a potential case, act quickly to insure that you obtain a signed consent from the patient and all the information, images, photographs, and samples you will need in order to write a thorough report. The consent form will be required by the journal. Check with the public relations professional at your institution. You will probably need to ask the patient to sign an institution media release giving you permission to take photos and present the case in a professional publication or at a professional conference. Some data will only be available for a short period of time. Collection of tissue samples and cultures may need to precede antibiotic treatment. Photos must be taken before the rash is treated or the swelling goes down. You cannot have too much data, but you can end up with missed opportunities if you fail to act in a timely fashion. Make sure the medical record is complete and you have all the data you will need for a good report.

As with a research report, one of the first steps in preparing a case report is to select a journal. Some journals rarely publish case reports. Look through recent issues of the journals you are considering and study a few case reports to get a sense of what the editor expects. Obtain the Author's Instructions from the selected journal's website and read it carefully. Comply with each instruction precisely. Case reports usually include an introduction, a case, and a discussion.

Introduction

The introduction should include a brief description of the disorder, incidence/prevalence, and an explanation for why it is important to study this case. A historical perspective may be added. The introduction is usually a short overview of the general disorder, with a limited number of references.

The Case

The case is structured like a case presentation. Begin with a description of the person, followed by a discussion of the presenting circumstances. Describe the physical examination and the laboratory results. Provide normal laboratory values for less commonly ordered tests. Discuss any images (x-rays, CT, or MRI). Outline the treatment and the results. If the treatment outcome was unusual, contrast it with the expected outcomes. Describe the follow-up.

Discussion

The discussion will require you to perform a thorough literature search that reveals any research findings or previous reports related to the unusual aspects of your case. Explain why your case is unique. A concise overview of the pertinent literature is appropriate, but remember, a case report is meant to be short. You are not writing a review article. Case reports are usually limited to fewer than 1500 words and five to 15 references.

The discussion ends with a conclusion. This is where you emphasize what lessons are to be learned from the case. You might encourage physicians to be vigilant and to recognize certain disorders if a particular set of symptoms occur. The author can make recommendations in the conclusion.

End the case report with your bibliography. The same submission and review process is used for a case report as an original article.

Some Final Suggestions

Many of us suffer from Blank Page Paralysis. Getting started on a writing project is hard. You don't have to write the introduction first. The methods may be an easier place to start. Try getting an outline saved on your computer, and then go back and make sentences or paragraphs out of the words or phrases in your outline. As additional topics come to mind that you want to discuss, add them to your outline. Don't worry too much about getting every word just right or keeping the length down when you write the first draft. It is easy to get rid of the chaff when all the nuggets are clearly in view. Understand, too, that the first version is NOT the final version. Most of us go through revision after revision before we are willing to share our writing with anyone else. Writing improves with practice, and manuscripts usually improve with thoughtful revision.

The more colleagues, mentors, and collaborators who read a manuscript, the more likely you are to catch errors before they are sent to the journal editor. Ask your critics to point out the parts of your manuscript that they find confusing. Try not to be defensive; the harshest critic will probably be the greatest help to you in improving your manuscript.

When a project is finally complete and an investigator has actually found the time to write it up for publication, there is a tendency to want to send it off immediately. This is a good time to let the manuscript simmer. Hold it for a week and take a last look with 'fresh eyes.' The number of items you will correct/improve in that fresh reading will surprise you. Then read it one last time to correct any errors you caused in your last revision.

16 How to Survive and Thrive in the Peer Review Process

Kathleen Kendall-Tackett, PhD, IBCLC, FAPA

Submitting articles to peer-reviewed journals can be one of the most unpleasant aspects of academic life. Promotions, tenure, grants, and awards are all tied to getting articles through this process. The hard reality is that getting a journal article published is an uphill battle. A journal's prestige is based, at least in part, on the percentage of articles they reject. The higher the rejection rate, the more prestigious the journal, but even the most prestigious journal still needs to publish articles. They might as well be yours. The purpose of this chapter is to walk you through some of the ins and outs of peer-review, and how to survive or even thrive.

The most important function of peer review is quality control. Two or three sets of eyes on a paper increase the likelihood that errors will be spotted and corrected. Peer review helps editors deal with specialized topics beyond the limits of his/her own experience. Knowledgeable reviewers can assure the editor of the quality and validity of the work reported. Peer review also has the potential to identify research fraud, but it is far from fool proof. Outright fraud

205

is, fortunately, fairly rare. But peer review can help detect it. Finally, peer review is important for the author. Reviewers often provide useful feedback that assists in the production of an improved manuscript.

The Peer Review Process

The first step in mastering peer review is making wise choices about where to send your work. I always recommend that the authors identify the journal they plan to send their articles to before they even begin to write. Why? Because every journal is unique. "Not appropriate for the journal" is one of the most common reasons for rejection.

If the journal you select is not one you normally read, spend some time getting to know it. Read through a few back issues. Think about the audience. Who reads this journal? What do you need to tell them? Read through the instructions for authors. Also look at the articles themselves. What type of articles are they? Are they research, clinical, or a mix of both? Most journals develop a certain flavor, which means some articles are going to be more likely accepted than others.

The next step is to look at the structure of the articles. How long is the introduction and literature review? Some journals, particularly ones with a more clinical focus, tend to have very short literature reviews (typically one to two manuscript pages). Others, especially if they are more research/or theory oriented, tend to have more complicated literature reviews. Longer literature reviews are also more common when there are complex statistical models, such as structural equation modeling, multiple regression, or path analysis, as the authors must provide justification from previous studies for the model they use.

You should also scrutinize the Methods section. A mismatch here can doom your paper. Some journals want only experimental data, so don't send them a case report or a paper based on survey data. Don't submit an article using qualitative analyses if all the journal publishes is quantitative. And if they never publish complex statistical models, they probably won't publish yours either. Pay attention to the type of results they publish and how the discussion is used: as a separate section or combined with the results.

You should also know that some journals will never publish articles on topics where they have an opposing view. I've run into this several times when trying to get papers published on controversial topics, such as extended breastfeeding and mother-infant bedsharing. If a journal editor or the reviewers have strong views, it will be quite difficult to get an article published in that particular journal. That doesn't mean that you might not want to try it. They may surprise you by accepting your article. Alternatively, you may choose to not waste your time with the "rejection step" and send your article to a journal that might be more receptive.

Another factor is the overall writing style. While most want articles that are "professional," how that's defined varies a surprising amount. Some journals prefer articles that are written in a more academic (Read: "windbag") style. Other journals want more concise language, active construction of verbs, and a readable style. Journals with a more readable style are often aimed at clinicians, who frankly do not have time to wade through page upon page of pompous prose.

Another factor to consider is article length. More and more journals are instituting strict page or word counts. Exceed the page length at your peril. I have recently rejected several manuscripts because they were well over the normal length. While there can be some exceptions to this, remember, editors are *looking* for reasons to reject manuscripts. So don't hand them one.

Not all journals have "blind" review, which means the reviewers may know who you are. Reviewers are usually anonymous. Some journals offer the option of blind review, but many journals are moving in the direction of non-blinded reviews. If you are writing for a journal outside of your field, you may need someone on the author list who has the "right" credentials (e.g., if writing for a nursing journal, you may need at least one co-author who is a nurse).

Finally, do yourself a favor and learn to write well. I find that reviews that take the longest are those where the article has some merit (so can't be rejected out of hand), but is written so poorly that it's difficult to wade through. As someone who reads manuscripts for a living, and who has read thousands of manuscripts, I can tell you that a well-written manuscript stands out like a shiny coin in the mud. Reviewers are often so thrilled by good writing that they tend to be more positive about your article overall. That being said, writing well can be a challenge, especially if you are writing in your non-native language. If this is a concern, you might consider finding a native speaker to collaborate with.

If you are in doubt about whether a journal might be a good match for your article, contact the editor or editorial assistant and ask whether your paper might be appropriate for their journal.

Submitting Your Article

Most well-established journals have electronic submission portals. You will upload your article into this online portal, which will collect information about you and your co-authors. It may also ask you for names of possible reviewers for your article. I've had students ask me how that could possibly be a good idea in that you might just list your friends and family.

It might be helpful if you see this process from the other side. When an article comes into an editor's work box via the electronic submission system, the editor then assigns reviewers for the article. Before I assign reviewers, I read the title and abstract, and briefly read the manuscript. I then search our database for reviewers with expertise on the topic. I generally assign three to five reviewers for a given manuscript. If it is a fairly specialized topic and not many potential reviewers appear, I will then look at the author's suggestions. I obviously won't send a manuscript to someone with the same last name as the author, or who is even part of the author's institution (although in a couple of cases, I've made exceptions if it's a highly specialized topic and no other choices were available). Generally speaking, the peer review process relies, to a certain extent, on the honor system. So part of the process from the editorial side involves trusting both the author and the reviewer to be professional and give an honest critique.

I may also decide to bring in a novice reviewer. For the journal *Clinical Lactation,* for example, I find it helpful to get feedback from clinicians who do not know the topic. Since my reviewer represents the final reader of the article, these reviewers can often identify areas where the author has not been clear.

Making the Decision

Once an editor receives reviews, the next step is to make a decision about whether to publish the article. This is usually not a yes-no decision; there are various stages of "maybe" in between. For editors, this is often the most time-consuming part of the process. I read through the manuscript, the reviews, and the Score Sheets, where reviewers rate various technical aspects of the manuscript and make a publication recommendation. These Score Sheets also list any confidential comments that reviewers make to the editors about the manuscript (see Figure 16.1).

Clinical Lactation

Official Journal of the United States Lactation Consultant Association

Ms. # [NUMBER]

Reviewer [NUMBER]

Score Sheet

Evaluation	High	Medium	Low
Significance of the manuscript			
Appropriateness of content for CL			
Quality of design/ methodology			
Quality of the writing			

Recommendation

Publish as is	
Publish with minor revision	
Publish with major revision	
Revise and resubmit	
Reject	

Confidential Comments to the Editor (List Below)

Figure 16.1. Sample Score Sheet

If your manuscript is rejected, you are free to send it someplace else.

"Accept as is" is another straightforward response. Not surprisingly, this response is quite rare. I've had only two articles accepted this way: one of mine, and one written with one of my students. I told her not to ever expect to see one of those again.

Most manuscripts fall into the "maybe" category, also known as "revise and resubmit." In this category, an editor can:

- Accept pending minor revisions
- Accept pending major revisions
- Reject with the option to resubmit

There are varying levels of "revise and resubmit." Some have "strong encouragement" to resubmit (Figure 16.2). If the editor asks for you to complete your revision within a specific period of time (e.g., six weeks), that is a particularly good sign.

Dear [AUTHOR]:

Thank you for submitting your manuscript titled [TITLE] to *Clinical Lactation*. Enclosed please find the three responses of our reviewers. As you can see, they felt that the manuscript has merit but requires some revisions.

When you submit the revised version of the manuscript please include a cover letter identifying how you addressed each suggestion, where in the manuscript the revision can be found, or, if you feel the recommended change was not warranted, your rationale for not making it.

Your revised manuscript may be resent to the reviewers. I look forward to receiving the revised version of the manuscript. I would appreciate it if you can make the revisions and get the new version back to me at your earliest convenience.

With warm regards,

Kathleen Kendall-Tackett, PhD, IBCLC
Editor-in-Chief

Figure 16.2. Example of "Revise and Resubmit" Letter - Strong Likelihood of Acceptance for Publication

Other "revise and resubmits" are more tepid (more like "you can send this back if you want and we promise to not set it on fire"). Even with the latter response, you can still get your paper published if you respond appropriately to the critiques the reviewers made.

Responding to a Revise and Resubmit

Learning to respond to "revise and resubmit" letters is every bit as important as writing a good paper in the first place. This is where your skill in negotiating can make a difference. Some reviews will be helpful, and some will be downright rude. Don't let rude comments derail you. You must handle reviewers' comments in an orderly and respectful manner.

There are two components to your response: the letter to the editor and the revised manuscript. Both are important, but the more critical component (and the part that many authors give short shrift) is the letter to the editor. When you submit the revised version of the manuscript include a cover letter identifying how you addressed each suggestion, where in the manuscript the revision can be found, or if you feel the recommended change was not warranted, your rationale for not making it.

Editors will use your cover letter to ensure that each of the reviewers' concerns was addressed. Don't skimp on this part. This is not the place for a cursory summary of the changes or the comment, "the changes were too numerous to name individually." Assume that the reviewers will see your letter and behave professionally. Go through the reviewers' advice and revise your manuscript in keeping with their suggestions when you agree with the feedback. It is a good idea to use a word processor tracking feature when you revise your manuscript or highlight your changes with a different colored font. Some journals will have specific instructions concerning the revisions. Make sure you follow them to the letter.

You do not need to go lock-step and make every change the reviewers suggested. Especially if there is more than one reviewer, their recommendations may contradict each other. Sometimes, a reviewer is wrong. In that case, you can cordially point out why you did not think the change was advisable. If you make a good case for ignoring the suggestion, the editor may agree, but realize that you can't do that with every point the reviewers made.

It is often a good idea to begin your response letter with a thank you. It never hurts to start nicely, and even if reviewers didn't get it right, they did give you a substantial chunk of their time. If nothing else, you can acknowledge that.

The next step is to systematically list each of the reviewer's points and explain how you revised the manuscript to conform with the suggestions, or why you did not alter your manuscript. This can be a lengthy and repetitive process, but the editor will look for a response to each reviewer comment. You can use a different font to indicate whether you are listing the reviewer's comment or your response (Figure 16.3).

Dear [Editor]:

Please find attached our revised manuscript entitled, [TITLE] that we resubmit for possible publication in [JOURNAL]. This manuscript reflects edits as suggested by the reviewers. We have also enclosed a point-by-point response to each of the reviewer's concerns.

Reviewer #1

1) The title and abstract should be changed to clearly indicate the hypothetical nature of the commitment.

We agree with the reviewer that the title and abstract of this manuscript do not clearly indicate the hypothetical nature of this study. Thus, the title has been changed to [TITLE]. The abstract has also been changed to clearly reflect this change.

2) The term "posttraumatic sequelae" should be changed to read "posttraumatic symptoms," or perhaps even better, "anxiety symptoms." There is no indication in these data that their symptoms are due to a sexual assault.

We agree that these symptoms are not necessarily due to the sexual assault by which this sample was screened. Thus, we changed "posttraumatic sequelae" to "posttraumatic symptoms." We elected to keep "posttraumatic" instead of replacing it with "anxiety" because we believe that depression, shame, and self-efficacy would not be accurately depicted with "anxiety symptoms."

Repeat for all the suggestions from each reviewer.

[AUTHOR] and I wish to thank you and the reviewers for the time you spent considering our manuscript and your many thoughtful and helpful comments. We feel that the current manuscript has been greatly strengthened, and we look forward to your response.

Sincerely yours,

Figure 16.3. Example of Revise and Resubmit Response

If Your Paper Is Rejected

Even the most seasoned researchers have articles rejected from time to time. Try not to take it personally. And don't make the mistake of discarding the paper. Go over the reviewers' comments with a more senior colleague who can help you weigh which comments are legitimate and which you can ignore. Before you make substantial revisions, think about which journal will receive your resubmission. Make the changes that you consider appropriate and that match the style of the new journal.

Can You Appeal a Decision?

In some cases, you may be able to appeal a rejection. Before you try, remember that this is not a time to be mouthy or belligerent. The editor is well within his or her rights to reject a manuscript based on the reviewers' feedback. However, it is sometimes possible to ask that the manuscript be sent to another reviewer.

Conclusions

It is possible to successfully navigate the peer-review system and publish in your field. The best approach is to do excellent work, submit your article to a journal that is a good match for your article, and to respond thoroughly to the reviewers' comments. If you do that, you dramatically improve your chances of getting your work out to the wider world.

References

Abbasi, A., Butt, N., Bhutto, A.R., Gulzar, K., & Munir, S.M. (2010). Hepatocellular carcinoma: A clinicopathological study. *Journal of the College of Physicians and Surgeons, 20*(8), 510-513.

Aitchison, J., Kay, J.W., & Lauder, I.J. (2005). *Interdisciplinary statistics: Statistical concepts and applications in clinical medicine.* Boca Raton, FL, USA: Chapman & Hall/CRC.

Alport, A.C. (1927). Hereditary familial congenital haemorrhagic nephritis. *British Medical Journal, 1*(3454), 504-506.

Anonymous. (2007). Biomedical research funding in FY 2008. *Physiologist, 50*(2), 67-68.

Aouizerate, J., Matignon, M., Kamar, N., Thervet, E., Randoux, C., Moulin, B., et al. (2010). Renal transplantation in patients with sarcoidosis: a French multicenter study. *Clinical Journal of the American Society of Nephrology, 5*(11), 2101-2108.

Armitage, P., & Berry, G. (1994). *Statistical methods in medical research* (3rd ed.). Oxford, UK: Blackwell Scientific Publications.

Baerlocher, M.O., O'Brien, J., Newton, M., Gautam, T., & Noble, J. (2010). Data integrity, reliability and fraud in medical research. *European Journal of Internal Medicine, 21*(1), 40-45.

Baliga, N.S. (2008). Systems biology. The scale of prediction. *Science, 320*(5881), 1297-1298.

Bankert, E.A.A., & Amdur, R.J. (2006). *Institutional Review Board: Management and Function* (2nd ed.). Sudbury, MA: Jones and Bartlett Publishers.

Baumslag, N. (2005). *Murderous medicine: Nazi doctors, human experimentation, and typhus.* Praeger Publishers.

Belle, G.V., Fisher, L.D., Heagerty, P. J., & Lumley, T. (2004). *Biostatistics: A methodology for the health sciences* (2nd ed.). Hoboken, NJ, USA: John Wiley & Sons.

Bennett, W.L., Gilson, M.M., Jamshidi, R., Burke, A.E., Segal, J.B., Steele, K.E., et al. (2010). Impact of bariatric surgery on hypertensive disorders in pregnancy: Retrospective analysis of insurance claims data. *BMJ, 340*, c1662. doi: 10.1136/bmj.c1662.

Bill and Melinda Gates Foundation. (2007). *Annual report. Grants paid summary.* Retrieved on September 12, 2011, from http://www.gatesfoundation.org/nr/public/media/annualreports/annualreport07/AR2007GrantsPaid.html.

Bjork, J., & Strömberg, U. (2005). Model specification and unmeasured confounders in partially ecologic analyses based on group proportions of exposed. *Scandinavian Journal of Work, Environment & Health, 31*(3), 184-190.

Bradley, M.C., Hughes, C.M., Cantwell, M.M., & Murray, L.J. (2010). Statins and pancreatic cancer risk: A nested case-control study. *Cancer Causes & Control, 21*(12), 2093-2100.

Brinkley, W.R. (1999). Disappearing physician-scientists. *Science, 283*(5403), 791.

Budd, J. M., Coble, Z.C., & Anderson, K.M. (2011). Retracted publications in biomedicine: Cause for concern. from http://www.ala.org/ala/mgrps/divs/acrl/events/national/2011/papers/retracted_publicatio.pdf.

Byrne, D.W. (1998). *Publishing your medical research paper. What they don't teach you in medical school.* Williams and Wilkins.

Caldwell, J.G., Price, E.V., Schroeter, A.L., & Fletcher, G.F. (1973). Aortic regurgitation in the Tuskegee study of untreated syphilis. *Journal of Chronic Diseases, 26*(3), 187-194.

Cameron, C., Chang, S., & Pagel, W. (2011). Scientific English: A program for addressing linguistic barriers of international research trainees in the United States. *Journal of Cancer Education, 26*(1), 72-78.

Canzonetta, C., Mulligan, C., Deutsch, S., Ruf, S., O'Doherty, A., Lyle, R., et al. (2008). DYRK1A-dosage imbalance perturbs NRSF/REST levels, deregulating pluripotency and embryonic stem cell fate in Down syndrome. *American Journal of Human Genetics, 83*(3), 388-400.

Chen, J.J., Lee, H.C., Yeung, C.Y., Chan, W.T., Jiang, C.B., & Sheu, J.C. (2010). Meta-analysis: The clinical features of the duodenal duplication cyst. *Journal of Pediatric Surgery, 45*(8), 1598-1606.

Cheng, A.Y., & Fantus, I.G. (2004). Thiazolidinedione-induced congestive heart failure. *The Annals of Pharmacotherapy, 38*(5), 817-820.

Claxton, L.D. (2005). Scientific authorship. Part 2. History, recurring issues, practices, and guidelines. *Mutation research, 589*(1), 31-45.

Cochrane Collaboration. (2011). *Glossary.* Retrieved on September 9, 2011, from http://www.cochrane.org/glossary.

Collins, F. (2010a). Opportunities for research and NIH. *Science, 327*(5961), 36-37.

Collins, F. (2010b). Statement for hearing entitled, "NIH in the 21st century: The director's perspective.Retrieved on September 12, 2011, from http:// www.nih.gov/about/director/budgetrequest/fy2011directorsperspective. pdf.

COS. (2011). COS funding opportunities. *Community of Science.* Retrieved on September 12, 2011, from http://fundingopps.cos.com/.

Coughlin S.S., & King, J. (2010). Breast and cervical cancer screening among women in metropolitan areas of the United States by county-level commuting time to work and use of public transportation, 2004 and 2006. *BMC Public Health, 10*, 146.

Crompton, J.G., Pollack, K.M., Oyetunji, T., Chang, D.C., Efron, D.T., Haut, E.R., et al. (2010). Racial disparities in motorcycle-related mortality: An analysis of the National Trauma Data Bank. *American Journal of Surgery, 200*(2), 191-196.

Daniel, W.W. (2009). *Biostatistics: A foundation for analysis in the health sciences* (9th ed.). Hoboken, NJ, USA: John Wiley & Sons, Inc.

Davis, M.S., Riske-Morris, M., & Diaz, S.R. (2007). Causal factors implicated in research misconduct: Evidence from ORI case files. *Science and Engineering Ethics, 13*(4), 395-414.

DeAngelis, C. (1990). *An introduction to clinical research.* Oxford, UK: Oxford University Press.

Depoy E., & Gitlin, L.N. (1998). *Introduction to research: Understanding and applying multiple strategies* (2nd ed. Vol. 288). Saint Louis,MO: Mosby.

Dougherty, J.A., & Rhoney, D.H. (2001). Gabapentin: A unique anti-epileptic agent. *Neurological Research, 23*(8), 821-829.

Down, J.L.H. (1866). Observations on an ethnic classification of idiots. *London Hosp Clin Lect Rep, 3*, 259.

Durbin, C.G., Jr. (2004). How to come up with a good research question: Framing the hypothesis. *Respiratory Care, 49*(10), 1195-1198.

Egger, M., Smith, G.D., & Phillips, A.N. (1997). Meta-analysis: Principles and procedures. *BMJ, 315*(7121), 1533-1537.

Encyclopedia of Everyday Law. (2003). *Informed consent.* Retrieved on December 13, 2010, from http://www.enotes.com/everyday-law-encyclopedia/ informed-consent.

Eyesnck, H.J. (1978). An exercise in mega-silliness. *American Psychologist, 33,* 157.

Fanelli, D. (2009). How many scientists fabricate and falsify research? A systematic review and meta-analysis of survey data. *PLoS One, 4*(5), e5738.

Farrugia, P., Petrisor, B.A., Farrokhyar, F., & Bhandari, M. (2010). Practical tips for surgical research: Research questions, hypotheses and objectives. *Canadian Journal of Surgery, 53*(4), 278-281.

Federal Register. (2005). Public health service policies on research misconduct. Final rule. *Federal Register, 70*(94), 28369-28400. Retrieved on September 12, 2011, from http://ori.dhhs.gov/documents/FR_Doc_05-9643.shtml.

Fleming, A. (1945). Nobel lecture – Penicillin. Retrieved on September 12, 2011, from http://nobelprize.org/nobel_prizes/medicine/laureates/1945/fleming-lecture.pdf.

Food and Drug Administration. (2011). CFR – Code of federal regulations title 21. Retrieved on September 13, 2011, from http://www.accessdata.fda.gov/scripts/cdrh/cfdocs/cfCFR/CFRSearch.cfm.

Foody, J.M., Farrell, M.H., & Krumholz, H.M. (2002). β-blocker therapy in heart failure. *JAMA, 287*(7), 883-889.

Foucault, M. (1994). *The birth of the clinic. An archaeology of medical perception.* New York: Random House.

Foundation Center (2011). Locate charitable funders for nonprofit organizations. Retrieved on September 9, 2011, from http://foundationcenter.org/findfunders/.

Framingham Heart Study. (2011). History of the Framingham Heart Study. Retrieved on September 9, 2011, from http://www.framinghamheartstudy.org/about/history.html.

Fuentes, J.J., Pritchard, M.A., Planas, A.M., Bosch, A., Ferrer, I., & Estivill, X. (1995). A new human gene from the Down syndrome critical region encodes a proline-rich protein highly expressed in fetal brain and heart. *Human Molecular Genetics, 4*(10), 1935-1944.

Gadomski A, de Long, R., Burdick, P., & Jenkins P. (2005). Do economic stresses influence child work hours on family farms? *J Agromedicie, 10*(2), 39-48.

Galie, N., Ghofrani, H.A., Torbicki, A., Barst, R.J., Rubin, L.J., Badesch, D., et al. (2005). Sildenafil citrate therapy for pulmonary arterial hypertension. *The New England Journal of Medicine, 353*(20), 2148-2157.

Gardner, W., Lidz, C.W., & Hartwig, K.C. (2005). Authors' reports about research integrity problems in clinical trials. *Contemporary Clinical Trials, 26*(2), 244-251.

Gilad, Y., Rifkin, S.A., & Pritchard, J.K. (2008). Revealing the architecture of gene regulation: The promise of eQTL studies. *Trends in Genetics, 24*(8), 408-415.

Glass, G.V. (1976). Primary, secondary, and meta-analysis of research. *Educational Researcher, 5*(10), 3-8.

Goldstein, J.L., & Brown, M.S. (2009). The LDL receptor. *Arteriosclerosis, Thrombosis, and Vascular Biology, 29*(4), 431-438.

Grace, S., & Higgs, J. (2010). Integrative medicine: Enhancing quality in primary health care. *Journal of Alternative and Complementary Medicine, 16*(9), 945-950.

Greenhalgh, T. (2010). Why did the Lancet take so long? *BMJ, 340*, c644.

Greenland, S., & Morgenstern, H. (1989). Ecological bias, confounding, and effect modification. *International Journal of Epidemiology, 18*(1), 269-274.

Gross, P.A. (1984). Collection of data documenting risk factors: Safeguards in conducting case-control studies. *The American Journal of Medicine, 76*(5A), 28-33.

Gruman, J., & Prager, D. (2002). Health research philanthropy in a time of plenty: A strategic agenda. *Health Affairs, 21*(5), 265-269.

Gunsalus, C.K., & Rennie, D. (2008). Handling whistleblowers: Bane and boon. In F. F. Wells & M. Farthing (Ed.), *Fraud and misconduct in biomedical research* (4th ed.). UK: Royal Society of Medicine Pr Ltd.

Hamilton, R. (2009). Agriculture's sustainable future: Breeding better crops. *Scientific American Earth, 19*(2), 16-17.

Hanefeld, M., & Belcher, G. (2001). Safety profile of pioglitazone. *International Journal of Clinical Practice. Supplement*(121), 27-31.

Harman, K., Bassett, R., Fenety, A., & Hoens, A. (2009). "I think it, but don't often write it": The barriers to charting in private practice. *Physiotherapy Canada, 61*(4), 252-258.

Haynes, R.B., Sackett, D.L., Guyatt, G.H., & Tugwell, P. (2006). *Clinical epidemiology: How to do clinical practice research* (3rd ed.). Philadelphia: Lippincott Williams Wilkins.

Hemphill, B. (2009). *Oral presentations.* Retrieved on September 9, 2011, from http://www.etsu.edu/scitech/langskil/oral.htm.

Henderson, G.E., Churchill, L.R., Davis, A.M., Easter, M.M., Grady, C., Joffe, S., et al. (2007). Clinical trials and medical care: Defining the therapeutic misconception. *PLoS Medicine, 4*(11), e324.

Hillman, G.C., Hedges, R., Moore, A., Colledge, S., & Pettitt, P. (2001). New evidence of late glacial cereal cultivation at Abu Hureyra on the Euphrates. *The Holocene, 11*(4), 383-393.

Hines, P.J., Wible, B., & McCartney, M. (2010). Learning to read, reading to learn. *Science, 328*(5977), 447.

Hoen, W.P., Walvoort, H.C., & Overbeke, A.J. (1998). What are the factors determining authorship and the order of the authors' names? A study among authors of the Nederlands Tijdschrift voor Geneeskunde (Dutch Journal of Medicine). *JAMA, 280*(3), 217-218.

Hulley, S.B., Cummings, S.R., Browner, W.S., Grady, D.G., & Newman, T.B. (2007). *Designing clinical research* (3rd ed., vol. 2). Philadelphia: Lippincott Williams Wilkins.

Iannelli, V. (2009). Vaccine preventable illnesses. Retrieved on September 9, 2011, from http://pediatrics.about.com/od/immunizations/a/0408_im_illness.htm.

ICMJE. (2009). Uniform requirements for manuscripts submitted to biomedcial journals: Ethical considerations in the conduct and reporting of research: Authorship and contributorship. Retrieved on September 12, 2011, from http://www.icmje.org/ethical_1author.html.

Jaffer, U., & Cameron, A.F.. (2006). Deceit and fraud in medical research. *International Journal of Surgery, 4*(2), 122-126.

Kaiser, J. (2008). NIH urged to focus on new ideas, new applicants. *Science, 319*(5867), 1169.

Kesselheim, A.S., Studdert, D.M., & Mello, MM. (2010). Whistle-blowers' experiences in fraud litigation against pharmaceutical companies. *New England Journal of Medicine, 362*(19), 1832-1839.

Kim, K., Zakharkin, S.O., & Allison, D.B. (2010). Expectations, validity, and reality in gene expression profiling. *Journal of Clinical Epidemiology, 63*(9), 950-959.

Kluge, E.H.W. (2007). Informed consent in health research: A practical guide for the global setting. *International Journal of Pharmaceutical Medicine, 21*(6), 405-414.

Koh, G.C., Wong, T.Y., Cheong, S.K., Lim, E.C., Seet, R.C., Tang, W.E., et al. (2010). Acceptability of medical students by patients from private and public family practices and specialist outpatient clinics. *Annals of the Academy of Medicine, Singapore, 39*(7), 555-510.

Korenberg, J.R. (1993). Toward a molecular understanding of Down syndrome. *Progress in Clinical and Biological Research, 384*, 87-115.

Lago, R.M., Singh, P.P., & Nesto, R.W. (2007). Congestive heart failure and cardiovascular death in patients with prediabetes and type 2 diabetes given thiazolidinediones: A meta-analysis of randomised clinical trials. *Lancet, 370*(9593), 1129-1136.

Lancet Editorial. (2008). The Wellcome Trust: An unsung hero in health research. *The Lancet, 371*(9612), 531-531.

Lebovitz H.E., Dole, J.F., Patwardhan, R., Rappaport, E.B., & Freed, M.I. (2001). Rosiglitazone monotherapy is effective in patients with type 2 diabetes. *The Journal of Clinical Endocrinology and Metabolism, 86*(1), 280-288.

Lejeune J., Gautier, M., & Turpin R. (1959). Etude des chromosomes somatiques de neuf enfants mongoliens. *Comptes Rendes de l'Académie des Sciences, 248*, 1721-1722.

Leroy, J.L., Habicht, J.P., Pelto, G., & Bertozzi, S.M. (2007). Current priorities in health research funding and lack of impact on the number of child deaths per year. *American Journal of Public Health, 97*(2), 219-223.

Lipowski, E.E. (2008). Developing great research questions. *American Journal of Health-System Pharmacy, 65*(17), 1667-1670.

Lipsey, M.W., & Wilson, D.B. (2001). *Practical meta-analysis.* Thousand Oaks, CA, USA: Sage Publications.

Liu, L., Zhuang, W., Wang, R.Q., Mukherjee, R., Xiao, S.M., Chen, Z., et al. (2011). Is dietary fat associated with the risk of colorectal cancer? A meta-analysis of 13 prospective cohort studies. *European Journal of Nutrition, 50*(3), 173-184.

Mackway-Jones, K. (2003). Seeking funding for research. *Emergency Medicine Journal, 20*(4), 359-361.

Manolio, T.A., & Collins, F.S. (2009). The HapMap and genome-wide association studies in diagnosis and therapy. *Annual Review of Medicine, 60*, 443-456.

Martinson, B.C., Anderson, M.S., & de Vries, R. (2005). Scientists behaving badly. *Nature, 435*(7043), 737-738.

Mascalzoni, D., Hicks, A., Pramstaller, P., & Wjst, M. (2008). Informed consent in the genomics era. *PLoS Medicine, 5*(9), e192.

McCoy, D., Kembhavi, G., Patel, J., & Luintel, A. (2009). The Bill & Melinda Gates Foundation's grant-making programme for global health. *The Lancet, 373*(9675), 1645-1653.

Medical News Today. (2006). *90% cure rate for acute lymphoblastic leukemia within reach.* Retrieved on September 12, 2011, from http://www.medicalnewstoday.com/releases/36106.php.

Mekdeci, B. (2011). Bendectin – How a commonly used drug cased birth defects. *Birth Defects Research for Children, Inc.* Retrieved on September 12, 2011, from http://www.birthdefects.org/research/bendectin_1.php.

Michalek, A.M., Hutson, A.D., Wicher, C.P., & Trump, D.L. (2010). The costs and underappreciated consequences of research misconduct: A case study. *PLoS Medicine, 7*(8), e1000318.

Morrow, R. (1989). A school-based program to increase seatbelt use. *The Journal of Family Practice, 29*(5), 517-520.

Moses, H., Dorsey, E.R., Matheson, D.H.M., & Thier, S.O. (2005). Financial anatomy of biomedical research. *JAMA, 294*(11), 1333-1342.

NIH DPCPSI. (2011). *Trans-NIH research: Scientific collaboration for the 21st century.* Retrieved on September 12, 2011, from http://opasi.nih.gov/collaboration/.

NIH. (2009). Enhancing peer review: The NIH announces enhanced review criteria for evaluation of research applications received for potential FY 2010 funding. *Center for Scientific Review.* Retrieved on September 12, 2011, from http://grants.nih.gov/grants/guide/notice-files/not-od-09-025.html.

NIH. (2010). Guidelines. Committee on Science Conduct and Ethics. Retrieved on September 12, 2011, from https://www.citiprogram.org/Default.asp?

NIH. (2008). Responsible conduct of research. *Bioethics resources on the web.* Retrieved on September 9, 2011, from http://bioethics.od.nih.gov/researchethics.html.

NIH. (2011a). *Funding opportunities & notices search results.* Office of Extramural Research. Retrieved on September 9, 2011, from http://grants.nih.gov/grants/guide/search_results.htm?year=active&scope=rfa.

NIH. (2011b). Glossary & acronym list - grant descriptions. Retrieved on September 12, 2011, from http://grants.nih.gov/grants/glossary.htm#R11.

Norman, G., & Streiner, D. (2009). *Statistics: The bare essentials* (3rd ed.). New York, USA: BC Decker.

Ogunyemi, D., Solnik, M.J., Alexander, C., Fong, A., & Azziz, R. (2010). Promoting residents' professional development and academic productivity using a structured faculty mentoring program. *Teaching and Learning in Medicine: An International Journal, 22*(2), 93-96.

ORI. (2008). *Annual Report.* Retrieved on September 12, 2011, from http://ori.hhs.gov/documents/annual_reports/ori_annual_report_2008.pdf.

ORI. (2010b). *Handling misconduct – Administrative actions.* Retrieved on September 9, 2011, from http://ori.dhhs.gov/misconduct/admin_actions.shtml.

ORI. (2010a) Tools - Plagiarism detection resources. Retrieved on September 12, 2011, from http://ori.hhs.gov/tools/plagiarism.shtml.

ORI. (1995). *ORI guidelines for institutions and whistleblowers: Responding to possible retaliation against whistleblowers in extramural research* (1995). Retrieved on September 12, 2011, from http://ori.hhs.gov/misconduct/Guidelines_Whistleblower.shtml.

ORI. (2009). *ORI policy on plagiarism.* Retrieved on September 12, 2011, from http://ori.hhs.gov/policies/plagiarism.shtml.

Panacek, E. (2007, May). Clinical research: Getting started. *Society of Academic Emergency Medicine Conference,* Chicago.

Pedroni, J.A., & Pimple, K.D. (2001). A brief introduction to informed consent in research with human subjects. Retrieved on September 12, 2011, from http://poynter.indiana.edu/sas/res/ic.pdf.

Petrie, A., & Watson, P. (1999). *Statistics for veterinary and animal sciences* (1st ed.). Oxford, UK.: Blackwell Publishing.

Perlman, D. (2004). Ethics in clincal research: A history of human subject protections and practical implementation of ethical standards. Retrieved on May 3, 2011, from http://www.socra.org/pdf/200405_Ethics_Clinical_Research_History.pdf.

Piantadosi, S., Byar, D.P., & Green, S.B. (1988). The ecological fallacy. *American Journal of Epidemiology, 127,* 893-904.

Portney, L.G., & Watkins, M.P. (2009). *Foundations of clinical research: Applications to practice* (3rd ed.). 2009. Upper Saddle River, NJ, USA: Pearson Education.

Pryor, E.R., Habermann, B., & Broome, M.E. (2007). Scientific misconduct from the perspective of research coordinators: A national survey. *Journal of Medical Ethics, 33*(6), 365-369.

Ravera, S., van Rein, N., de Gier, J.J., & de Jong – van den Berg, L.T.W. (2011). Road traffic accidents and psychotropic medication use in the Netherlands: A case-control study. *British Journal of Clinical Pharmacology, 72*(3), 505-513.

Renz, L., & Atienza, J. (2006). International grantmaking update: A snapshot of US foundation Trends. Retrieved on September 12, 2011, from http://foundationcenter.org/gainknowledge/research/pdf/intl_update_2006.

Research. (2011). *Find funding opportunities.* Retrieved on September 12, 2011, from http://www.researchresearch.com/.

Rosner, H., Rubin, L., & Kestenbaum, A. (1996). Gabapentin adjunctive therapy in neuropathic pain states. *The Clinical Journal of Pain, 12*(1), 56-58.

Rosoff, A. (2008). *Informed consent: A guide for health care providers.* Rockville, MD: Aspen Publishers.

Rubin, D.J., & McDonnell, M.E. (2010). Effect of a diabetes curriculum on internal medicine resident knowledge. *Endocrine Practice, 16*(3), 408-418.

Ruggles, C.L.N. (2005). *Ancient astronomy: An encyclopedia of cosmologies and myth.* Santa Barbara: ABC-Clio, pp. 354-355.

Rutecki, G.W. (2007). How much do we care when truth replaces fiction? Ethical conduct and human subjects research in Africa. *Center for Bioethics & Human Dignity.* Retrieved on September 12, 2011, from http://cbhd.org/content/how-much-do-we-care-when-truth-replaces-fiction-ethical-conduct-and-human-subject-research-a.

Schwartz, J. (2001). Oversite of human subject research: The role of the States. Retrieved on September 12, 2011, from http://www.onlineethics.org/Topics/RespResearch/ResResources/nbacindex/%20nbachindex/hschwartz.aspx.

Selvan, V., Vasylyeva, T.L., Turner, C., & Regueira, O. (2008). One disease, multiple manifestations. *Pediatric Annals, 37*(2), 92-95.

Shelledy, D.C. (2004). How to make an effective poster. *Respiratory Care, 49*(10), 1213-1216.

Silverman, H. (2007). Ethical issues during the conduct of clinical trials. *Proceedings of the American Thoracic Society, 4,* 180-184.

Simon, G.E., Unutzer, J., Young, B.E., & Pincus, H.A. (2000). Large medical databases, population-based research, and patient confidentiality. *The American Journal of Psychiatry, 157*(11), 1731-1737.

Sims, S., Willberg, C., & Klenerman, P. (2010). MHC-peptide tetramers for the analysis of antigen-specific T cells. *Expert Review of Vaccines, 9*(7), 765-774.

Slavin, R.E. (1986). Best-evidence synthesis: An alternative to meta-analytic and traditional reviews. *Educational Researcher, 15,* 5-11.

Steneck, N.H. (2011). *ORI introduction to the responsible conduct of research.* Retrieved on September 12, 2011, from http://ori.dhhs.gov/education/products/RCRintro/.

Texas Statutes. (2009). Search term – informed consent. Retrieved on September 15, 2011 from http://www.statutes.legis.state.tx.us/.

Thomson, C.A. (2007). Funding nutrition research: Where's the money? *Nutrition in Clinical Practice, 22*(6), 609-617.

U.S. Department of Health & Human Services. (2009). Code of Federal Regulations. Title 45. Public welfare. Part 46. Protection of human subjects. Retrieved on September 12, 2011, from http://www.hhs.gov/ohrp/humansubjects/guidance/45cfr46.html.

U.S. Department of Health & Human Services. (2011b). *Grant information for current and prospective HHS grantees.* Retrieved on September 9, 2011, from http://dhhs.gov/asfr/ogapa/aboutog/grantsnet.html.

U.S. Department of Health & Human Services. (2011a) Activity codes search results - Types of grants listed. Office of Extramural Research. Retrieved on September 12, 2011, from http://grants.nih.gov/grants/funding/ac_search_results.htm.

Van de Vijver, M.J., He, Y.D., van't Veer, L.J., Dai, H., Hart, A.A., Voskuil, D.W., et al. (2002). A gene-expression signature as a predictor of survival in breast cancer. *New England Journal of Medicine, 347*(25), 1999-2009.

Van Eaton, E.G., McDonough, K., Lober, W.B., Johnson, E.A., Pellegrini, C.A., & Horvath, K.D. (2010). Safety of using a computerized rounding and sign-out system to reduce resident duty hours. *Academic Medicine, 85*(7), 1189-1195.

Wadman, M. (2007). Biomedical philanthropy: State of the donation. *Nature, 447*(7142), 248-250.

Wakefield, J., & Haneuse, S.J. (2008). Overcoming ecologic bias using the two-phase study design. *American Journal of Epidemiology, 167*(8), 908-916.

Walker, A.E. (1942). Lissencephaly. *Archives of Neurology and Psychiatry, 48,* 13-29.

Warburg, M. (1971). The heterogeneity of microphthalmia in the mentally retarded. *Birth Defects Original Article Series, 7*(3), 136-154.

Weintraub, A.Y., Levy, A., Levi, I., Mazor, M., Wiznitzer, A., & Sheiner, E. (2008). Effect of bariatric surgery on pregnancy outcome. *International Journal of Gynaecology and Obstetrics, 103*(3), 246-251.

Wells, F., & Farthing, M.. (2008). *Fraud and misconduct in biomedical research* (4th ed.). UK: Royal Society of Medicine Pr Ltd.

Western Culture Global. (2009). The top 100 heroes of western culture. Retrieved on September 12, 2011, from http://westerncultureglobal.org/knowledge-philosophy.html.

Woollen, S.W., & Hage, A.E. (2001). Scientific misconduct – The "f" word. Retrieved on September 12, 2011, from http://www.pbelow-consulting.com/pdf/f_word_woollen_elhage_1001.pdf.

Index

A

Absolute risk reduction 125
Accuracy 82
- Addition rule 117
Administrative support 178
Adverse event 44, 96
Alternative hypothesis 118
Analysis of variance 122
ANOVA 122
Appendices 103
Arithmetic mean 112
Autonomy 86

B

Background 100
Background/needs assessment/
  rationale 155
Bar-graph 110
Before-after study 32, 82
Belmont Report 39, 86
Beneficence 86
Better treatment 94
Bias 73
Bimodal 113

Biological significance 121
Blank page paralysis 204
Blinding techniques 74
Budget 158

C

Case-control study 25, 81
Case report 21, 202
Case series 22
Categorical variables 112
Causal relationship 128
Children - research subjects 55
Chi-square test 123
Clinical importance 121
Clinical research 166
Clinical sensitivity 132
Clinical trial medicine 64
Clinical trial phases 67
Clinical trials 30
Clinical trial study 63
Clinical vignette abstract 187
Code book 107
Coefficient of variation 116
Cohort study 27, 81
Conditionally probable 118

Confidence interval 131
Conflict of interest 97
Consents within consents 91
Consequences of misconduct 148
Consumables 178
Continuing reviews 43
Continuous variables 112
Control subjects 73
Correlation coefficient 124, 127
Cronbach's Alpha 82
Cross-over trial 82
Cross-sectional studies 23, 81
Curative dose 79

D

Data collection 105
Data management 103
Declaration of Helsinki 86
Descriptive statistics 110
Descriptive study title 100
Diagnostic tests 132
Direct costs 158
Disclosure of errors 92
Discontinuous variables 112
Discussion 200, 203
Documentation 59
Dose escalation studies 77
Dot-plot 110

E

Ecological study 24
Eligibility requirements for funding
    181
Equipment 178
Ethical research 15
Ethics 85
Executive summary 154
Experimental design and methods
    157
Experimental studies 29

F

Fabrication 142
Falsification 142
Federal regulations 51

FINER 12
Focus groups 33
Food, Drug, and Cosmetic Act 63
Fraud 141
Frequency distribution 110
Full disclosure 96
Funding 177
Funding sources 153, 179, 181

G

Generic drugs 71
Geometric mean 113
Grant components 154
Grant opportunities 182
Grant success 172

H

Hazard rate 127
Hazard ratio 124, 127
Health Insurance Portability and
    Accountability Act 45
Heterogeneity management 79
Hippocratic Oath 86
Histogram 110
Hybrid study 27
Hypotheses 100, 118

I

Incidence 82
Incidence rate 124
Independent review 87
Indirect costs 159
Inferential statistics 117
Informed consent 49, 87, 88, 95
Institutional Review Board 37
Instructions for journal articles 196
Integrity of data 95
Inter-quartile range 114
Introduction 203
Introduction/background 198
Introductory summary 100
Investigators 100
IRB make-up 40

J

Journal selection 196
Justice 86
Justification 100

K

Kaplan-Meier survival analysis 129
Kasselbaum-Kennedy Act of 1996 45

L

Latin Square design 76
Legal age 92
Letter to the editor 212
Limitations of proposed research 160
Linear regression 128
Line-graph 110
Literature review 10
Logistic regression 128
Longitudinal cohort study 27
Longitudinal study 81

M

Mann-Whitney U test 120, 131
Material and methods 101
Measurement of association 124
Measures of central tendency 112
Measures of dispersion 112, 113
Median 113
Mentor 10
Meta-analysis review 136
Meta-analysis study 28
Methods 198
Missing data points 107
Mode 113
Monitoring 70
Multiplication rule 118

N

Nested case-cohort study 27
Nested case-control study 27
NIH review process 163
NIH structure 167
Nominal variable 112
Nonmalficence 86

Normal distribution 118
Null hypothesis 118
Nuremberg Code 86

O

Objectives 100
Observational study 19, 81
Odds ratio 124
One-sample t-test 120
One-tailed test 119
Oral presentation 186, 190
Ordinal variables 112

P

Paired t-test 120
Parental rights 89
Peer-review process 205
Personnel and environment 156
Philanthropic funding 179
PICOT 11
Pie-charts 110
Plagiarism 142, 146
Poster presentation 186, 191
Precision 82
Pre-clinical research 64
Predictive value 132
Pregnant women - research subjects
57
Prevalence 82
Prisoners - research subjects 58
Probability 117
Probability distribution graph 118
Product recalls 70
Proof reading 201
Prospective study 27, 80
Protection of privacy 94
Protocol amendment 44
Protocol deviations 43
Publication in peer-reviewed journals
195

Q

Quasi-random trial 32

R

Randomization 73
Randomized controlled study 30
Randomized controlled trial 82
Randomized cross-over clinical trials 31
Range 114
Ratio of probability 124
Receiver operating characteristic (ROC) curves 133
References 103, 160, 200
Regression 128
Relative risk 124
Relative risk reduction 125
Relevance 16
Reliability 82
Reporting fraud 147
Research abstract 186, 188
Research grant funding success 182
Research idea 152
Research question 10
Research support 178
Results 199
Retrospective study 27, 80
Revise and resubmit 212
Revision of manuscript 201
Right to withdraw 96
Risk-benefit ratio 77
Risk factors 124
Risks 103
Risks vs. benefits 96
Rules for grant writing 153

S

Safeguards for a well-designed study 145
Scatter diagram 110
Scientific presentations 185
Sigmoidal curve 78
Source of Supplies 93
Spearman's rank correlation coefficient 128
Staff 178
Standard deviation 115
Standard error of the means 116

Statement of closure 44
Statistical analysis 103
Statistical package 108
Statistical significance 121
Statistical software 137
Statistics 109
Student's t-test 120
Study design 19, 35
Study protocol 99
Study team design 66
Survival analysis 129
Systematic review 136

T

Tenets of clinical research 87
Time series study 27
Timetable 159
Translational research 34, 163
Trial designs 74
Two-sample t-test 120
Two-tailed test 119
Type I error 120
Type II error 121

U

Unimodal 113
Use of subject's tissues 97

V

Validity 82
Variance 114

W

Wards of the State - research subjects 56
Welch's t-test 120
Wilcoxon rank sum test 131

Editor Bio

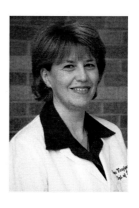

Tetyana L. Vasylyeva, MD, PhD, Doctor of Medical Science (Ukraine), is a Professor in the Department of Pediatrics, Nephrology Section, at Texas Tech University Health Sciences Center in Amarillo, Texas. She has dedicated her life to improving children's health, both as a practicing pediatrician and as a researcher.

Dr. Vasylyeva began her career in the Ukraine, earning an MD, PhD and Doctor of Medical Science, which is the highest academic research degree awarded in a number of countries including Ukraine. After immigrating to the U.S., she worked her way up the professional ladder by completing a post-doctoral fellowship, pediatric residency, and nephrology fellowship.

As a professor at Texas Tech University Health Sciences Center, Dr. Vasylyeva has established a new nephrology service for the Panhandle area, where she cares for children with renal disease, acute and chronic renal injury, and end stage renal disease. She is on the staff at Northwest Texas Healthcare System and Baptist St. Anthony's Health System.

Dr. Vasylyeva is passionate about medical research and directs her efforts toward 'bench to bedside' translational research. She is the principal investigator on multiple projects, has a translational research laboratory, and has active ongoing clinical studies.

Ordering Information

Hale Publishing, L.P.
1712 N. Forest Street
Amarillo, Texas, USA 79106

8:00 am to 5:00 pm CST

Call » 806.376.9900
Toll free » 800.378.1317
Fax » 806.376.9901

Online Orders
www.ibreastfeeding.com